Disclaimer Notice:
Please note the information contained within this document is for educational and entertainment purposes only. All effort has been executed to present accurate, up to date, reliable, complete information. No warranties of any kind are declared or implied. Readers acknowledge that the author is not engaged in the rendering of legal, financial, medical, or professional advice. The content within this book has been derived from various sources. Please consult a licensed professional before attempting any techniques outlined in this book.

By reading this document, the reader agrees that under no circumstances is the author responsible for any losses, direct or indirect, that are incurred as a result of the use of the information contained within this document, including, but not limited to, errors, omissions, or inaccuracies.

CONTENTS

Introduction

The contents that you are about to feast your eyes on I am sure will spark a new light in you that you as a diabetic never thought you would feel again! While there are many things that diabetics cannot consume, there is none of that negativity here! All of the smoothies within the chapters of this book are great for everyone, many harboring ingredients that can actually *improve* your health as one with this ever-growing disease.

For those that don't know too much about green smoothies and what makes them so healthy, it's important to gain some knowledge as to all the good, healthy ingredients you will be whipping up in your blender in the near future!

3 Steps for a Perfect Diabetic-Friendly Smoothie

1. **Pick three servings of produce – 2 fruits, 1 green**
   - *Per serving of fruit – ½ C*
   - *Per serving of greens – 1 C*
2. **Pick one serving of liquid (and add ice to fill)**
   - *1 C of liquid per smoothie*
3. **Pick up to two servings of protein or fiber**
   - 1 tablespoon per smoothie

Tips on Green Smoothie Creation

- ***Keep Proportions in Check*** – When it comes to whipping up green smoothies that will treat you right, proportion are everything. Try to stick to 40% greens and 60% other ingredients. Greens add the biggest impact in nutritional value, but if you use them to a greater extent your smoothie will taste like a nasty, liquefied salad.
- ***Easy on the fruit*** – When first starting out, many experiment with combining different food flavors to find a niche that satisfies their taste buds. 2-3 fruits are quite plenty for any one smoothie combination. If you go adding all the produce to a blender, you will more than likely not enjoy the outcome taste-wise.
- ***Be creative!*** – While you should keep in mind what you are throwing into your blend to mix, do not be afraid of trying new ingredients and strong flavor combinations. You may be surprised at what you come up with!
- ***Make it yours*** – Even though there are loads of ingredients in this book to get you started, if there are ingredients you enjoy or that fit your lifestyle better, by all means, utilize them! Everyone has different tastes and texture preferences. Make sure YOU enjoy it!
- ***Walk on the wild side of green*** – Even though it is recommended that you blend only 1-2 green ingredients with several fruits, do not be hesitant to visit outside that boundary. There are many combinations of

veggies that if blended together, can make for quite a bright, happy tasting smoothie!

Green Smoothie Facts

- Strawberries, blackberries and blueberries are high in fiber and antioxidants, which assists in preventing cardiovascular diseases, cancer and other chronic illnesses.
- Women should consume up to 45 grams of carbohydrates per smoothie, as men should aim for 60 grams of carbs per smoothie.
- Spinach contains alpha-lipoic acid, which greatly influences lower triglycerides and weight loss in those with Type 2 Diabetes.
- Coconut water contains l-arginine, which helps reduce concentrations of blood glucose in diabetics.
- Adding protein and fiber to smoothie assists in the slowing of glucose absorption in the bloodstream.
- Peanut butter actually is very beneficial for diabetics, in that it helps moderate glucose concentrations and aids in controlling appetite.

There are plenty of books that discuss recipes to fuel a diabetic's body on the market, thanks again for choosing this one! Every effort was made to ensure it is full of as many scrumptious smoothie recipes as possible for you to sip on! Please enjoy!

Chapter 1: Berry Blast

#1 Berry Green Smoothie

218.7 Calories – 49.7g Carbs – 1.7g Fat – 34.3g Sugar – 4.7g Protein
1 T stevia, 2 T old fashioned oats, ½ C milk, 1 ripe banana, ½ C frozen strawberries, ½ C frozen blueberries, 1 C spinach leaves.
Combine all ingredients in a blender until smooth.

#2 Mixed Berry Green Smoothie

136 Calories – 26g Carbs – 0.1g Fat – 19.1g Sugar – 9.9g Protein
1 C frozen unsweetened mixed berries, ½ C + 2 T nonfat milk, and 2 C baby spinach.
Blend and pulse all of the ingredients until smooth, scraping sides when needed. Enjoy!

#3 Wild Blueberry Citrus Green Smoothie

319 Calories – 23.3g Carbs – 2.3g Fat – 12.1g Sugar – 33.1g Protein
2 Cs frozen spinach, ½ small grapefruit, ½ C orange, 1 frozen banana, 2 T vanilla protein powder, 1.5 Cs unsweetened almond milk.
Blend all ingredients until creamy.

#4 Basic Berry Smoothie

287 Calories – 15.4g Carbs – 3.7g Fat – 11.3g Sugar – 12.4g Protein
1 C spinach, 1.5 Cs frozen berry of choice, 2 T rolled oats, 1 C almond milk, ½ banana.
Blend all ingredients and top with a banana slice and/or frozen berries.

#5 Basic Berry with Kale

Replace spinach with Kale.

#6 Cherry Nut Smoothie

264 Calories – 10.9g Carbs – 2.9g Fat – 12.9g Sugar – 9.4g Protein
1 C spinach, 1.5 Cs frozen cherries, 2 T nut butter of choice, 1 C almond milk, and ¼ t vanilla extract.
Mix up everything until well combined and slightly frothy. Top with frozen cherry.

#7 Blueberry and Avocado Detox Green Smoothie

290 Calories – 11g Carbs – 6.4g Fat – 11g Sugar – 6.9g Protein

1-2 Cs coconut water, 1 handful spinach, 1 cucumber, 1 C frozen blueberries, 1 frozen banana, 1 avocado.

Blend ingredients until silly smooth.

#8 Go-Go Goji Berry Smoothie

207 Calories – 39g Carbs – 5g Fat – 23g Sugar – 6g Protein

1 C ice, ½ C water, 2 T goji berries, 2 T sunflower seeds, 2 peeled oranges, 1.5 Cs chopped carrots, 1 C kale.

Blend components of smoothie until you reach desired texture.

#9 Camu Camu Berry Berry Smoothie

108 Calories – 24g Carbs – 2g Fat – 14g Sugar – 3g Protein

½ C ice, 1 C water, 1 T flaxseed, 1 t camu camu powder, 1 pitted nectarine, 1.5 Cs mixed berries, 1 handful Swiss chard.

Combine ingredients until smooth in texture.

#10 Cacao Maqui Grape

248 Calories – 27g Carbs – 13g Fat – 14g Sugar – 7g Protein

½ C ice, 1 C water, 1 T raw cacao, 1 t maqui powder, ½ C raw cashews, 1 C red grapes, 1-2 handfuls baby romaine.

Incorporate ingredients together until combined. Top with red grape halves.

#11 Blueberry Carrot Smoothie

76 Calories – 11g Carbs – 0g Fat – 7.5g Sugar – 3g Protein

10 baby carrots, ½ C orange juice, 2 Cs water, handful spinach or kale, 2 Cs frozen blueberries.

Combine all ingredients together until well blended and smooth.

#12 Blueberry Pomegranate Smoothie

67 Calories – 8g Carbs – 0g Fat – 4g Sugar – 2g Protein

1 frozen banana, 1 C spinach, ½ C pomegranate juice, 1 C frozen blueberries.

Blend everything until silky and/or frothy.

#13 Mixed Berry Coconut Water Smoothie

101 Calories – 18g Carbs – 3g Fat – 12g Sugar – 3g Protein

1 T flax seed meal, 1 C fresh spinach, 2 Cs frozen mixed berries, 2 Cs coconut water frozen into ice cubes.

Pour in components of smoothie and blend on high until smooth and creamy.

#14 No-Banana Berry Green Smoothie

202 Calories – 23g Carbs – 4g Fat – 14.5g Sugar – 3g Protein

½ C orange juice, ½ C plain Greek yogurt, ½ C frozen raspberries, ½ C frozen strawberries, 1 C baby spinach.

Blend all ingredients on high until you reach desired smoothness.

#15 Double Green Goddess Smoothie

117 Calories – 12g Carbs – 0.3g Fat – 2g Sugar – 33.2g Protein

1-2 handfuls ice, ½ avocado, ½ cucumber, ½ green pear, ½ green apple, 1 kiwi fruit, 1 stalk celery, ¾ C spinach, 1 scoop vanilla protein powder, 1 C ice cold water.

Combine the ingredients within the blender, pulsing on high until frothy and creamy.

#16 Berry Banana Breakfast Smoothie

332 Calories – 77g Carbs – 3g Fat – 12g Sugar – 4g Protein

1 C almond milk, 1 chopped apple of choice, ½ C frozen raspberries, ½ C frozen blueberries, ½ C frozen strawberries, 1 frozen banana.

Combine all ingredients until smooth and creamy. Top with any additional frozen berries.

#17 Get Your Greens Berry Smoothie

190 Calories – 19g Carbs – 3g Fat – 12g Sugar – 2g Protein

1.5 Cs frozen cherries or mixed berries, 1.5 Cs baby spinach, 1.5 Cs milk of choice.

Blend all ingredients until nice and creamy.

Chapter 2: Fruit-full Delights

#18 Green Mango Smoothie

231 Calories – 11.3g Carbs – 9.9g Fat – 12g Sugar – 9.8g Protein

1 C spinach, 1.5 Cs frozen mango, ¼ C Greek yogurt, 1 C water, and ¼ C freshly grated ginger.

Combine components in a blender on high until smooth.

#19 Green Peach Smoothie

248 Calories – 12g Carbs – 2.7g Fat – 12.7g Sugar – 8.4g Protein

1 C spinach, 1.5 Cs frozen peach, 2 T hemp, 1 C coconut water, ¼ t ground cinnamon.

Blend all ingredients until silky. Top with a pinch of cinnamon.

#20 Green Peach with Kale

Replace spinach with kale.

#21 Pina Colada Smoothie

265 Calories – 11.3g Carbs -3.3g Fat – 15.4g Sugar – 7.8g Protein

1 C spinach, 1.5 Cs frozen pineapple, 1 T chia seeds, 1 C coconut water, 1 T shredded coconut.

Blend everything until frothy. Top with pineapple slice.

#22 Pina Colada with Kale

Replace spinach with Kale

#23 Extremely Green Smoothie

228 Calories – 12g Carbs – 3.9g Fat – 14g Sugar – 5.6g Protein

½ apple of choice, juice of 1 lemon, 1 C spinach, 1 C kale, ½ C cucumber, ½ C cilantro, 1 C coconut water, 1 T hemp seeds.

Blend all components until combined. Garnish with extra hemp seeds.

#24 Mango Mint Green Smoothie

268 Calories – 9.1g Carbs – 3.3g Fat – 14.6g Sugar – 9.5g Protein

½ lime juiced, ¼ C mint leaves, ½ C Greek yogurt, ½ C almond milk, ½ C frozen mango, 2 Cs spinach.

Blend until all is smooth in texture. Serve chilled.

#25 Mango Mint Green with Kale
Replace spinach with Kale.

#26 Happy Digestion Smoothie
304 Calories – 10.9g Carbs – 4.9g Fat – 15.9g Sugar – 10g Protein
¼ t probiotic powder (optional), 1 t freshly grated ginger, 2 T avocado, ¼ C fresh parsley leaves, ½ C coconut water, ½ C water, ½ frozen banana, 1 C frozen pineapple.
Blend all ingredients until combined and super smooth.

#27 Pineapple Lemon Parsley Green Smoothie
118 Calories – 31g Carbs – 1g Fat – 18g Sugar – 5g Protein
5 drops liquid stevia, 2 C frozen pineapple, 2 peels and seeded lemons, 1 handful of chopped parsley, ½ cucumber, ¾ C coconut water.
Combine everything until thoroughly blended. Enjoy!

#28 Zesty Orange Zucchini Smoothie
103 Calories – 21g Carbs – 2g Fat - 15g Sugar – 3g Protein
1 C ice, 1.5 Cs coconut water, 1 T flax seed, ½ t turmeric, ½ juiced lemon, 1 orange, 1 yellow zucchini, 1.5 Cs kale.
Blend ingredients until smooth in texture.

#29 Zesty Orange Zucchini with Spinach
Replace kale with spinach or baby spinach.

#30 Pear Ginger Wheatgrass Smoothie
54 Calories – 12g Carbs – 0g Fat – 7g Sugar – 1g Protein
1 C ice, 1 C water, 1/8 ounce wheatgrass, ½ inch ginger, 1 pear, 1 handful green romaine.
Blend all ingredients until you reach your desired texture.

#31 Orange Rosemary Pomegranate

77 Calories – 12g Carbs – 3g Fat – 7g Sugar – 3g Protein

1 C ice, ½ C water, 1 sprig of fresh rosemary, 1 T hemp seed, 1 t pomegranate powder, 1 peeled orange, 2 handfuls baby kale.
Blend until silky smooth.

#32 Sweet Bok Choy

76 Calories – 20g Carbs – 0g Fat – 15g Sugar – 1g Protein

1 handful ice, 1 C water, 1 chopped apple of choice, ½ juiced lemon, 1 peeled orange, 1-2 handfuls bok choy.
Combine everything in a blender on high until silky.

#33 Blueberry Fig Smoothie

101 Calories – 19g Carbs – 3g Fat – 14g Sugar – 3g Protein

½ C ice, 1.5 Cs water, 1 T hemp seed, 2 figs, ½ C frozen blueberries, 1-2 handfuls romaine lettuce.
Blend all ingredients until well combined. The color may not be pleasing the eye but the taste sure is to your taste buds!

#34 A Sage Pear

59 Calories – 15g Carbs – 0g Fat – 9g Sugar – 1g Protein

1 C ice, 1 C water, ½ t moringa, 1 sprig of sage, ½ juiced lemon, 1 chopped pear, 1-2 handfuls chard.
Blend until you reach desired consistency. Top with extra moringa.

#35 Sage Pear with Spinach

Replace chard with spinach or baby spinach.

#36 Apple Crisp Smoothie

184 Calories – 28g Carbs – 7g Fat – 14g Sugar – 5g Protein

1 C ice, 1 C water, 1 t baobab powder, ¼ C raw cashews, ¼ C gluten free oats, 1 chopped apple of choice, ½ C grapes of choice, 2 handfuls baby romaine.
Blend ingredients together until you achieve smooth texture and darkish green color.

#37 Apple Crisp with Spinach

Substitute baby romaine for spinach or baby spinach.

#38 Spicy Apple Cabbage Smoothie

201 Calories – 27g Carbs – 10g Fat – 16g Sugar – 5g Protein

1 C ice, 1 C water, 2 T goji berries, ¼ C walnuts, 1 juiced lemon, 1 chopped apple of choice, 2 leaves of cabbage.

Mix ingredients together until mainly smooth in texture.

#39 A Pear of Beets

153 Calories – 19g Carbs – 7g Fat – 12g Sugar – 5g Protein

1 C ice, 1 C water, 1 T hemp seed, 2 T almonds, ½ inch ginger, 1 chopped pear, 1 C chopped beets, 1 C spinach.

Blend everything in a blender on high until you reach a smooth, brightly beet colored mixture. Top with extra almonds.

#40 Pear of Beets with Kale

Replace spinach with kale or baby kale.

#41 Orange Beet Mixer

103 Calories – 20g Carbs – 2g Fat – 13g Sugar – 3g Protein

1 C ice, 1 C water, 1 T chia seeds, ½ inch ginger, ½ C frozen blueberries, 1 peeled orange, 1 beet, 1 bunch of baby spinach.

Mix components together to create a purple-ish in color smoothie mixture.

#42 Cardamom Peach Smoothie

85 Calories – 20g Carbs – 1g Fat – 9g Sugar -3g Protein

1 C ice, 1 C water, 1/8 t cardamom, 1 T white mulberries, ½ C cantaloupe, 1 peach, 1-2 handfuls chard.

Mix ingredients together until well combined.

#43 Cardamom Peach with Spinach

Replace chard with spinach or baby spinach.

#44 Cardamom Peach with Kale
Replace chard with kale or baby kale.

#45 Blueberry Plum Basil Smoothie
75 Calories – 15g Carbs – 2g Fat – 10g Sugar – 1g Protein
1 C ice, 1.5 Cs coconut water, 4 basil leaves, 1 T flaxseed, ½ C frozen blueberries, 1-2 handfuls chard.
Blend together to create a thick but smooth texture.

#46 Blueberry Plum Basil with Spinach
Replace chard with spinach or baby spinach.

#47 Apple Pineapple Express
115 Calories – 15g Carbs – 2g Fat – 12g Sugar – 2g Protein
1 C ice, 1 C water, 1 T chia seeds, ½ C fresh mint, 1 chopped apple of choice, ½ C frozen pineapple, 1-2 handfuls kale.
Blend until smooth in texture. Top with a spring of mint.

#48 Apple Pineapple with Spinach
Replace kale with spinach or baby spinach.

#49 Red Pepper Apple
92 Calories – 16g Carbs – 2g Fat – 11g Sugar – 2g Protein
½ C ice, 1 C water, ½ inch ginger, 1 T hemp seed, ½ juiced lemon, 1 apple of choice, 1 red bell pepper, 1 C baby spinach.
Combine ingredients in blender until thoroughly combined. Top with a lemon slice.

#50 Apple Carrot Top
100 Calories, 19g Carbs – 2g Fat – 11g Sugar – 2g Protein
½ C ice, 1 C water, 1 T sunflower seeds, ½ inch peeled ginger, 1 chopped apple of choice, 1 C chopped carrots, 1 handful carrot greens.
Mix all ingredients together until smooth in texture.

#51 Apple Carrot Top with a Kick

Add in ½ seeded jalapeño and a couple dashes of cayenne pepper to recipe above.

#52 Sweet Potato Smoothie

82 Calories – 16g Carbs – 2g Fat – 9g Sugar – 2g Protein

½ C ice, 1 C water, 1 T flaxseed, 1 peeled orange, ¼ C frozen strawberries, ½ of a raw sweet potato.

Incorporate ingredients together until thoroughly combined. Top with a strawberry slice if desired.

#53 4-Ingredient Mango Green Smoothie

299 Calories – 72g Carbs – 0g Fat – 51.2g Sugar – 1g Protein

¾ C unsweetened almond milk, 1 C baby spinach leaves, 1 ripe banana, and 1.5 Cs frozen mango chunks.

Blend all ingredients until you reach a smooth, silky texture.

#54 4-Ingredient Mango with Kale

Replace spinach with kale or baby kale.

#55 Green Peach Lassi Smoothie

100 Calories – 15g Carbs – 1.5g Fat – 11g Sugar – 6g Protein

4 t natural sweetener of choice, pinch of Cardamom, ¾ C plain Greek yogurt, 1 C baby spinach, 2 Cs unsweetened vanilla almond milk, 4 Cs frozen peach slices.
Blend ingredients well until you achieve thick, silky mixture.

#56 Pineapple Pomegranate Smoothie

209 Calories – 50g Carbs – 3g Fat – 36g Sugar – 4g Protein

½ C water, ½ C frozen raspberries, ¼ C pomegranate seeds, ½ C frozen pineapple, 1-2 handfuls spinach or kale.

Incorporate ingredients together until blended well.

#57 Orange Carrot Mango Smoothie

242 Calories – 59g Carbs – 0g Fat – 44g Sugar – 4g Protein

1 T lime juice, ¾ C frozen pineapple, ¾ C frozen mango, ½ C orange juice, ½ C carrot juice, 1-2 handfuls spinach.
Blend ingredients until well combined.

#58 Orange Carrot Mango with Kale
Replace spinach with kale or baby kale.

#59 Green Apple Smoothie
127 Calories – 23g Carbs – 4g Fat – 19g Sugar – 2g Protein
Pinch of nutmeg, ½ t cinnamon, 1 C ice, 1 C spinach, 2 Cs water, 2 granny smith apples, ¼ C dates.
Blend everything on high until smooth in texture.

#60 Green Apple with Romaine
Replace spinach with romaine or baby romaine lettuce.

#61 Cherry Almond Spinach Smoothie
138 Calories – 26g Carbs – 5g Fat – 21g Sugar – 2.5g Protein
1-2 Cs spinach, ¾ C orange juice, 1 frozen banana, 1 C frozen cherries, ¾ C water, ¼ C raw almonds. Optional: Chia seeds, hemp seeds, protein powder.
Mix ingredients together, blending until smooth in texture. Top with optional ingredients if desired.

#62 Super Green Back on Track Smoothie
146 Calories – 30g Carbs – 3g Fat – 24g Sugar – 2g Protein
2-3 whole limes, 2 Cs almond milk, 2-3 Cs greens of choice, 1.5 Cs frozen mango, 1.5 Cs frozen pineapple.
Combine ingredients on high until you reach desired consistency. Enjoy!

#63 Citrus Flax Green Smoothie
151 Calories – 30.9g Carbs – 3.4g Fat – 18.3g Sugar – 3.6g Protein
½ C frozen pineapple chunks, 2 T flaxseeds, 2 Cs spinach, 1 frozen banana, 2 peeled clementines, and ½ C water.
Blend components until smooth.

#64 Citrus Flax with Chard
Replace spinach with Swiss chard.

#65 Lime and Coconut Green Smoothie

178 Calories – 28g Carbs – 4g Fat – 14g Sugar – 4g Protein

Handful ice, 2 C spinach, ½ frozen banana, ½ C coconut water, ½ C coconut milk, juice of 1 lime.

Layer ingredients together within blender jar and pulse until smooth.

#66 Mango Cashew Smoothie

143 Calories – 26g Carbs – 2g Fat – 11g Sugar – 3g Protein

1 lime, 1 T chia seeds, 2 Cs almond milk, ½ C cashew nuts, 2 Cs spinach, 2 frozen bananas, 1 chopped mango.

Blend until creamy. Enjoy with a sprinkle of chia seeds.

#67 Pineapple Paradise Spinach Smoothie

250 Calories – 31.3g Carbs – 15g Fat – 17g Sugar – 3.8g Protein

½ C ice, 2 Cs spinach, 1 ripe avocado, 2 Cs pineapple chunks, ¾ C water.

Blend all ingredients until creamy. Top with a couple additional chunks of pineapple.

#68 Coconut Mango Green Smoothie

235 Calories – 29g Carbs – 11g Fat – 8g Sugar – 7g Protein

½ t flaked coconut, ½ C frozen mango, ½ t vanilla extract, 1 C coconut milk, 2 T chia seeds, 1 handful spinach leaves.

Blend until smooth and creamy.

#69 Orange Dream Green Smoothie

129 Calories – 25g Carbs – 0g Fat – 14g Sugar – 10g Protein

½ C ice, ¼ C plain Greek yogurt, ¼ C almond milk, 1 t honey, 1 t vanilla extract, 1 peeled orange, 1 handful spinach.

Blend until creamy and slightly frothy. Top with orange slice

#70 Creamy Chia Seed Pina Colada Smoothie

289 Calories – 24g Carbs – 15g Fat – 9g Sugar – 16g Protein

1 t coconut oil, 1 t flaked coconut, ½ C plain Greek yogurt, 1 C frozen pineapple chunks, 1 C coconut milk, 1 T chia seeds, 1 handful spinach.

Combine until creamy and top with a wedge of lime.

#71 Island Green Smoothie
198 Calories – 21g Carbs – 11g Fat – 10g Sugar – 11g Protein
1 C water, 1 handful kale, 1 handful spinach, ½ frozen banana, ½ C frozen pineapple chunks, ½ C frozen mango chunks, ¼ C turbinado sugar.
Blend until creamy.

#72 Pink Grapefruit Detox Smoothie
201 Calories – 19g Carbs – 7g Fat – 10g Sugar – 3g Protein
½ inch piece fresh ginger, 2 Cs fresh spinach, 4 large pink juiced grapefruits, 1 T chia seeds, 1 frozen banana, 2 C frozen or fresh pineapple chunks, ½ C baby spinach.
Combine all ingredients until smooth. Garnish with a quarter of a grapefruit wedge.

#73 Kiwi- Strawberry Green Smoothie
204 Calories – 25g Carbs – 4g Fat – 12g Sugar – 2g Protein
1.5 Cs ice, 2 T sweetener of choice, 1 C frozen strawberries, 2 peeled kiwi fruits, 1 C spinach.
Combine ingredients together until you reach desired texture.

Chapter 3: Banana-Rama

#74 Banana Nut Smoothie

278 Calories – 11.1g Carbs – 4.5g Fat – 18.2g Sugar – 7.8g Protein

1 C spinach, 1.5 Cs frozen banana, ¼ C nuts of choice, 1 C almond milk, 1 T cocoa powder.

Blend everything together until frothy. Top with chopped nuts and/or cocoa.

#75 Banana Nut Smoothie with Kale

Replace spinach with kale.

#76 Banana Mango Avocado Green Smoothie

357 Calories – 14.8g Carbs – 8.8g Fat – 13g Sugar – 10g Protein

Few drops of stevia, splash of vanilla extract, 1 C almond milk, ½ avocado, 1 C spinach, 1 C frozen mango chunks, 1 frozen banana.

Blend ingredients until smooth in texture.

#77 Banana Mango Avocado with Kale

Substitute spinach with kale or baby kale.

#78 Strawberry Banana Green Smoothies (In a Bag!)

249 Calories – 31g Carbs – 6g Fat – 15g Sugar – 22g Protein

For pre-prepared bags – 4 t chia seeds, 4 Cs spinach, 2 Cs whole strawberries, 2 Cs sliced bananas. *For Blending* – ½ - 1 C unsweetened almond milk, 1 scoop vanilla protein powder.

Taking 4-quart freezer bags, add 1 C frozen fruit, 1 handful spinach and 1 t chia seeds to each. Then put in freezer. When ready to blend, add almond milk and protein powder and pulse until you reach the consistency you desire.

#79 Strawberry Banana with Kale

Replace spinach with kale or baby kale.

#80 Strawberry Banana with Collard Greens

Replace spinach with collard greens.

#81 Kids-Friendly Green Smoothie

115 Calories – 11g Carbs – 7.5g Fat – 12.3g Sugar – 3g Protein

1 T chia seeds, 1.5 Cs frozen pineapple, 1 C frozen mango, 1 frozen banana, 1.5 Cs spinach or kale, 1.5 – 2 Cs water, ½ C coconut milk.

Blend until you reach desired consistency, adding more water if needed. Your kids are sure to sip soundly on this one!

#82 Banana Mango Smoothie

103 Calories – 8g Carbs – 5g Fat – 10g Sugar – 2g Protein

1 T honey, 1.5 – 2 Cs skim milk, ½ frozen banana, 1-2 Cs frozen mango, ½ C spinach or kale.

Blend until creamy.

#83 Banana Kiwi Smoothie

291 Calories – 38g Carbs – 2g Fat – 22g Sugar – 34g Protein

1 t stevia, 1 scoop protein powder of choice, ½ frozen banana, 1 sliced kiwi fruit, ¾ C plain Greek yogurt, handful spinach or kale.

Mix components of smoothie until well blended.

#84 Glowing Skin Smoothie

156 Calories – 29g Carbs – 3g Fat – 17g Sugar – 4g Protein

½ sliced avocado, 2 Cs spinach or kale, 1 C frozen mango chunks, 1 C frozen pineapple, 2 ripe/frozen bananas, ½ C coconut water, and 1 T ground flax.

Blend until combined. Top with additional flax seeds if desired.

#85 Banana Peach Spinach Smoothie

130 Calories – 23g Carbs – 2g Fat – 19g Sugar – 3g Protein

½ C Greek yogurt, 2 handfuls spinach, splash of orange juice, 2 peaches, 1 frozen banana.

Blend everything on high until smooth.

#86 Banana Peach Kale
Replace spinach with kale or baby kale.

#87 Banana Peach Chard
Replace spinach with Swiss chard.

#88 Banana Peach Romaine
Replace spinach with romaine or baby romaine lettuce.

#89 Banana, Chocolate and Almond Butter Smoothie
151 Calories – 24g Carbs – 5g Fat – 2g Sugar – 3g Protein
1 handful ice, 1 T almond butter, 1 T fat free chocolate syrup, 1 frozen banana, 1 C unsweetened almond milk, 1 handful baby kale.
Blend until creamy.

#90 Banana Chocolate Almond with Spinach
Replace kale with spinach or baby spinach.

#91 Banana Chocolate Bacon Green Smoothie
278 Calories – 25g Carbs – 8g Fat – 1g Sugar – 5g Protein
Handful ice, 4 strips of cooked bacon, 1 frozen banana, 1 T honey, 1 T cocoa powder, ½ C spinach, 1 C coconut milk.
Blend components of smoothie on high until creamy. Top with additional bacon if desired.

#92 Banana Chocolate Bacon with Chard
Replace spinach with Swiss chard.

#93 Banana Chocolate Bacon with Collard Greens
Replace spinach with collard greens.

Chapter 4: Melon Heaven

#94 Hydrating Lemon-Lime Cantaloupe Cooler

69 Calories – 11g Carbs – 2g Fat – 7g Sugar – 3g Protein

1 C ice, 1 C water, 1 T chia seeds, 1 t Natural Calm, ½ lime juiced, 1 C cantaloupe, 2 handfuls baby kale.

Blend components until you reach a smooth-like texture.

#95 Lemon-Lime Cantaloupe with Spinach

Substitute kale with spinach or baby spinach.

#96 Pumpkin Seed Cantaloupe

80 Calories – 11g Carbs – 3g Fat- 9g Sugar – 6g Protein

1 C ice, 1 C water, 1 T pumpkin seed, 4-6 strawberries, 1 C cantaloupe, 2 handfuls baby spinach.

Blend until well combined.

#97 Pumpkin Seed Cantaloupe with Kale

Substitute spinach for kale or baby kale.

#98 Watermelon Mint Smoothie

81 Calories – 13g Carbs – 2g Fat – 7g Sugar – 2g Protein

½ C ice, 1 C water, 1 T hemp seed, 6 sprigs mint, 1.5 Cs watermelon, 2 cucumbers, 1 C kale.

Blend all ingredients until combined thoroughly. Refresh your taste buds by adding a sprig of mint when consuming.

#99 Watermelon Mint with Spinach

Substitute kale for spinach or baby spinach.

#100 Honey Rose Petal Smoothie

121 Calories – 20g Carbs – 4g Fat – 15g Sugar – 3g Protein

1 C ice, 1 C water, 1 T pistachios, 2 rose buds, ½ C frozen strawberries, 1.5 Cs honeydew, 1-2 handfuls spinach.

Blend until nice and smooth.

#101 Lavender Honey Smoothie

116 Calories – 26g Carbs – 2g Fat – 18g Sugar – 3g Protein

½ C ice, 1.5 Cs coconut water, 1 T chia seeds, ¼ t lavender, ½ C frozen blueberries, 1 C honeydew, 1-2 handfuls spinach.

Blend ingredients until smooth. I promise this smoothie tastes better than it appears! Sprinkle with chia seeds and enjoy!

#102 Lavender Honey with Kale

Substitute spinach for kale or baby kale.

#103 Cucumber Cantaloupe

75 Calories – 11g Carbs – 3g Fat – 7g Sugar – 3g Protein

½ C ice, 1 C water, 2 sprigs mint, 1 T hemp seed, ½ juiced lime, 1 C cantaloupe, 1 cucumber, 1-2 handfuls spinach.

Incorporate components of smoothie until smooth. Top with hemp seeds.

#104 Cucumber Cantaloupe with Chard

Substitute spinach for Swiss chard.

#105 Like Bees to Honey(dew)

48 Calories – 11g Carbs – 0g Fat- 8g Sugar – 2g Protein

½ C ice, 1 C water, 1 t bee pollen, 2 sprigs mint, 1 pitted peach, ½ C honeydew, 1-2 handfuls collard greens.

Combine everything in a blender on high speed until frothy.

#106 Like Bees to Honeydew with Spinach

Replace collard greens with spinach of baby spinach.

#107 Like Bees to Honeydew with Kale

Substitute collard greens with kale or baby kale.

#108 Refreshing Cucumber Melon Smoothie

59 Calories – 2g Carbs – 0g Fat – 4.5g Sugar – 1g Protein

1 C water, 1 C ice, ½ honeydew melon, 1 cucumber, handful spinach.

Blend all until well combined and a bit frothy in texture.

#109 Refreshing Cucumber Melon with Romaine

Substitute spinach with romaine or baby romaine lettuce.

#110 Cool n' Creamy Cantaloupe Smoothie

98 Calories – 4g Carbs – 1g Fat – 2g Sugar – 1g Protein

1 C ice, 2 T honey, 1 C plain Greek yogurt, 1 chopped cantaloupe, 1 C kale.
Blend all ingredients together until combined.

#111 Watermelon Mojito Smoothie

70 Calories – 2g Carbs – 0g Fat – 2.5g Sugar – 1g Protein

Handful ice, juice of 1 lime, 8 leaves of mint, ¼ large watermelon, and 1-2 small handfuls spinach.
Blend all ingredients until you achieve a nice and smooth mixture. Serve with a sprig of mint.

#112 Summertime Blast Smoothie

182 Calories – 47g Carbs – 1g Fat – 5g Sugar – 3g Protein

4-5 fresh basil leaves, 2/3 C ice, ¼ C frozen pineapple, 1 frozen banana, ½ of a chopped frozen cantaloupe, 2 t lemon juice, 2/3 C seedless watermelon, ½ C baby spinach.
Blend components until frothy. Enjoy this refreshing drink!

#113 Summertime Blast with Chard

Substitute spinach for Swiss chard.

#114 Mango Melon Madness Green Smoothie

156 Calories – 32g Carbs – 0g Fat – 3g Sugar – 2.5g Protein

1.5 Cs diced melon, 1.5 C frozen mango chunks, 2 Cs cold coconut water, 2 Cs fresh spinach leaves.
Blend spinach with coconut water first, then add remaining ingredients to blender, pulsing until smooth.

#115 Mango Melon Madness with Kale

Substitute spinach with kale or baby kale.

#116 Honeydew Melon Smoothie
129 Calories – 28g Carbs – 1g Fat – 2g Sugar – 4g Protein
2 Cs skim milk, ½ C vanilla Greek yogurt, ½ C fresh baby spinach, 2 Cs frozen honeydew.
Blend until combined and smooth.

#117 Honeydew Melon with Kale
Replace spinach with kale or baby kale.

#118 Mighty Melon Green Tea Smoothie
160 Calories – 24g Carbs – 2g Fat – 5g Sugar – 3g Protein
4 fresh mint leaves, ½ C plain Greek yogurt, 1 chopped pear, 1 C cantaloupe, 1 C frozen pineapple chunks, 1 C brewed green tea of choice, ½ C spinach.
Place all ingredients in blender and pulse until smooth.

#119 Summer Melon Smoothie
201 Calories – 23g Carbs – 1g Fat – 11g Sugar – 4g Protein
1/8 t ground ginger, 1.5 Cs watermelon chunks, 1.5 Cs cantaloupe chunks, 1 frozen banana, 2 Cs frozen strawberries, ½ C kale.
Blend until combined.

#120 Cantaloupe Smoothie
214 Calories – 24g Carbs – 2.6g Fat – 6g Sugar – 24.6g Protein
1-2 Cs ice, 2-4 T gelatin, 1 C Greek yogurt, 2 Cs cantaloupe, 1 C spinach.
Create gelatin by box, then add it in with remaining ingredients, blending until creamy.

#121 Strawberry Cantaloupe Smoothie
201 Calories – 21g Carbs – 1.8g Fat – 4g Sugar – 19g Protein
1 T chia seeds, 1 t honey, 1 frozen banana, 1 cantaloupe, 1 C frozen strawberries, ½ C milk of choice, ½ C romaine lettuce.
Combine ingredients until smooth. Top with strawberry slice.

#122 Minty Melon Smoothie
157 Calories – 19g Carbs – 0.7g Fat – 2g Sugar – 12g Protein
1 C ice, 10 mint leaves, ¼ C lime juice, 2 T honey, 2/3 C vanilla Greek yogurt, 1.5 Cs honeydew melon, 1 C kale.
Blend components until combined and smooth in texture. Garnish with a mint leaf.

#123 Peach Cantaloupe Smoothie

179 Calories – 15g Carbs – 1g Fat – 4g Sugar – 5.6g Protein

½ C ice, ½ T honey, ¾ C light peach yogurt, 4 slices frozen peaches, 1 C ripe cantaloupe, ½ C baby spinach.

Blend until well incorporated and smooth.

#124 Kiwi Honeydew Melon Smoothie

190 Calories – 20g Carbs – 2g Fat – 1.5g Sugar – 5g Protein

2 kiwi fruits, 1 C halved green grapes, 2 Cs honeydew melon, ¾ C vanilla Greek yogurt, ½ C spinach.

Blend ingredients together until you get a nice and creamy consistency.

#125 Blueberry Melon Smoothie

202 Calories – 26g Carbs – 7g Fat – 3g Sugar – 28g Protein

1 t ground flax seed, 1 scoop vanilla protein powder, ¼ C milk, ¾ C vanilla Greek yogurt, 1 C frozen blueberries, 1 C frozen cantaloupe, ½ C spinach.

Combine ingredients until creamy. Garnish with additional blueberries.

#126 Blueberry Melon with Chard

Replace spinach with Swiss chard.

#127 Blueberry Melon with Kale

Replace spinach with kale or baby kale.

#128 Raspberry Melon Smoothie

179 Calories – 28g Carbs – 5g Fat – 9g Sugar – 8.5g Protein

2 Cs agave nectar, 1 C baby spinach, ½ C vanilla Greek yogurt, ½ C frozen raspberries, 2 Cs frozen cantaloupe.

Blend until combined and creamy in texture. Garnish with additional raspberries.

#129 Raspberry Melon with Kale

Substitute spinach with kale or baby kale.

#130 Raspberry Melon with Romaine

Replace spinach with romaine or baby romaine lettuce.

Chapter 5: All Hale Kale

#131 Green Coconut Tonic Smoothie

279 Calories – 11g Carbs – 4.3g Fat – 17.3g Sugar – 7.3g Protein

1 T flaxseed meal, 1 C coconut water, 1" piece of ginger, ½ C lemon, ¼ C cilantro, ½ C cucumber, 1 C carrot, 2 Cs kale.

Blend all ingredients until combined, scraping blender jar as needed.

#132 Green Coconut Tonic with Spinach

Substitute kale with spinach or baby spinach.

#133 Pineapple Kale Smoothie

301 Calories – 9.9g Carbs – 8.3g Fat – 20.1g Sugar – 9g Protein

2 Cs raw kale, ¼ C frozen pineapple, ¾ C almonds, 1 frozen banana, ¼ C Greek yogurt, 2 T peanut butter, 1 T honey.

Blend everything on high speed until combined and smooth.

#134 Kale, Blueberry, Avocado and Mango Smoothie

341 Calories – 14g Carbs – 7.8g Fat – 13.9g Sugar – 10g Protein

1 C kale, 1.5 Cs frozen mango, 1 C frozen blueberries, ½ avocado, 1 T chia seeds, 1 t maca powder, 1 T honey, 2 T almond butter, 1.5 Cs coconut water.

Blend all ingredients together until you reach desired consistency.

#135 Lean Green Smoothie

275 Calories – 11g Carbs – 9g Fat – 8.3g Sugar – 10g Protein

1 T hemp seeds, 1-2 Cs water, 1 lime, ½ C green grapes, 10 mint leaves, 1-2 handfuls of kale.

Blend until smooth. Top with mint leaf.

#136 Lean Green with Spinach

Substitute kale with spinach or baby spinach.

#137 Lean Green Smoothie with Chard

Replace kale with Swiss chard.

#138 Green and Clean Machine Smoothie

281 Calories – 8.4g Carbs – 8.3g Fat – 3.4g Sugar – 11.9g Protein

1-2 Cs water, 1 T chia seeds, ½ green apple, 10 mint leaves, ¼ C cucumber, 2 celery stalks, 1-2 handfuls kale.

Blend until well combined. Top with mint leaf if desired.

#139 Katie's Kale Smoothie

311 Calories – 9g Carbs – 4.5g Fat – 12.9g Sugar – 8.3g Protein

½ pear, 1 orange, 2 Cs kale, 1 C grape of choice, ½ frozen banana.

Blend until you achieve a super smooth texture. Top with extra fruit.

#140 Kale Plum Crumble

262 Calories – 43g Carbs – 6g Fat – 37g Sugar – 5g Protein

1 C ice, 1 C water, 4 walnuts, 3 dates, 1/8 t cinnamon, 1/8 t nutmeg, ¼ C gluten free oats, ½ C frozen strawberries, 2 shiro plums, 1-2 handfuls kale.

Blend up all ingredients until smooth in texture. Feel free to garnish with nuts or a dash of cinnamon.

#141 Spinach Plum Crumble

Replace kale with spinach or baby spinach.

#142 Green Kale Lagerfeld

67 Calories – 16g Carbs – 0g Fat – 9g Sugar – 3g Protein

1 C water, ½ t spurulina, ½ juiced lemon, 1 Pink Lady apple, 1 cucumber, 1-2 handfuls kale.

Combine all ingredients in a blender, pulsing until you achieve texture you desire.

#143 Orange Beet Smoothie

54 Calories – 13g Carbs – 0g Fat – 9g Sugar – 1g Protein

½ C ice, 1 C water, ½ inch ginger, ½ juiced lemon, 1 peeled orange, 1 chopped beet, 1 C kale.

Blend together until nice and smooth in texture. Garnish with a lemon slice.

#144 Orange Beet with Spinach

Substitute kale with spinach or baby spinach.

#145 Orange Beet with Romaine

Substitute kale with romaine or baby romaine lettuce.

#146 Apples and Pears Green Smoothie

105 Calories – 23g Carbs – 2g Fat – 15g Sugar – 2g Protein

Handful ice, 1 C water, 1 T flaxseed, 1 chopped pear, 1 chopped apple of choice, 1-2 handfuls baby kale.

Blend components until combined.

#147 Maple Ginger Glazed Carrot Smoothie

127 Calories – 24g Carbs – 3g Fat – 16g Sugar – 3g Protein

1 C ice, 1 C water, 1 T hemp seed, 2 t real maple syrup, ½ inch ginger, 1 chopped apple of choice, 1/5 Cs chopped carrots, 1 handful carrot greens, 1 handful baby kale.

Blend ingredients until smooth.

#148 Ginger Cranberry Smoothie

121 Calories – 24g Carbs – 2g Fat – 13g Sugar – 4g Protein

1 C ice, ½ C water, 1 T chia seeds, ½ inch ginger, 2 peeled oranges, ¼ C cranberries, 1 cucumber, 1-2 handfuls baby kale.

Blend everything together until you reach desired consistency. Top with extra cranberries.

#149 Ginger Cranberry with Spinach

Replace kale with spinach or baby spinach.

#150 Ginger Cranberry with Chard

Replace kale with Swiss chard.

#151 Turmeric Carrot Smoothie

100 Calories – 19g Carbs – 3g Fat – 11g Sugar – 3g Protein

½ C ice, 1 C water, 1 t turmeric, 1 T sunflower seeds, ½ juiced lemon, 1 orange, 3 carrots, 1-2 handfuls baby kale.

Blend until smooth. Top with carrot shavings if desired.

#152 Carrot Coconut Lime Smoothie

119 Calories – 24g Carbs – 3g Fat – 13g Sugar – 2g Protein

1 C ice, 1.5 Cs water, 1 T shredded coconut, ½ juiced lime, 1 apple of choice, 3 medium carrots, 1-2 handfuls kale.

Blend ingredients until smooth in texture. Garnish with extra coconut.

#153 Cucumber Dill Smoothie
49 Calories – 8g Carbs – 2g Fat – 3g Sugar – 2g Protein
½ C ice cubes, ½ C water, 1 T pistachios, ½ juiced lemon, 5 sprigs of dill, 1 cucumber.
Incorporate components until they are completely blended. Top with a sprig of dill for looks if desired.

#154 Cucumber Dill with Spinach
Replace kale with spinach or baby spinach.

#155 Cucumber Dill with Romaine
Replace kale with romaine or baby romaine.

#156 Tropical Green Storm
67 Calories – 9.4g Carbs – 2.3g Fat – 3g Sugar – 2.9g Protein
½ C frozen or fresh pineapple, ½ C real orange juice, 1 C kale, ½ C almond milk, ½ C fresh or frozen mango, 1 T flax seed, agave nectar (to taste).
Blend ingredients until smooth. Garnish with a slice of pineapple if desired. Enjoy!

#157 Bone Broth Green Smoothie
112 Calories – 11.3g Carbs – 5g Fat – 1g Sugar – 7.5g Protein
½ t salt, 1 T coconut oil, 2 T lemon juice, 1/3 C cilantro, 1 C leeks, 3 Cs kale, 1.5 Cs chopped celery, 1 C chopped carrots, 4 Cs bone broth.
Sauté coconut oil in a sauce pan or instant pot. Allow time for oil to melt and add in carrots, sautéing them for 3-5 minutes. Add remaining veggies and salt, sautéing for a few minutes until softened. Then add bone broth and lemon juice. Simmer mixture for 25-30 minutes. Remove lid and allow mixture to cool down. Place in blender on high speed until combined. Serve chilled or warm.

#158 Bone Broth with Spinach
Replace kale with spinach or baby spinach.

#159 Strawberry Kale Smoothie

317 Calories – 24.9g Carbs – 8.3g Fat – 13g Sugar – 11.3g Protein
1.5 Cs non-dairy milk, ½ C frozen strawberries, ½ Cs kale, ½ frozen banana, 2 T hemp seeds, 2 Cs baby spinach.
Blend until smooth and creamy.

#160 Strawberry Spinach

Replace kale with spinach or baby spinach.

#161 Strawberry Chard

Replace kale with Swiss chard.

#162 The Super Kale Green Smoothie

190 Calories – 21g Carbs – 3g Fat – 11g Sugar – 3g Protein
¼ C chopped mint, ¼ C chopped parsley, 1 C orange juice, 2 stalks celery, 1.25 Cs frozen mango chunks, 1.25 Cs kale leaves.
Combine ingredients until frothy and creamy in texture.

#163 Ice Cream Kale Shake Smoothie

301 Calories – 31g Carbs – 5g Fat – 14g Sugar – 4g Protein
1 pinch sea salt, 1 t minced ginger, 1 t pure vanilla extract, 2 T chopped dates, ½ C raw cashews, ½ C water, 2 Cs ice, 2 frozen bananas, 1 C curly kale leaves.
Blend until extremely creamy, adding more ice if needed to achieve desired texture.

Chapter 6:Spinach Ain't Just for Popeye

#164 Anti-Inflammatory Spinach Smoothie

218 Calories – 8.3g Carbs – 3.4g Fat – 11g Sugar – 5.2g Protein

1 T flaxseed meal, 1 C coconut water, 1 t turmeric, 1" piece of ginger, ¼ C frozen berries of choice, 1 C frozen pineapple, 2 Cs spinach.

Blend all components until you achieve desired consistency.

#165 Low-Carb Smoothie

375 Calories – 4g Carbs – 25g Fat – 12.3g Sugar – 30g Protein

1 scoop protein powder, 10 drops liquid stevia, 1 T coconut oil, ¼ C avocado, ¼ C celery, ¼ C cucumber, 1 handful spinach, 1.5 Cs almond milk.

Blend all together until smooth in texture. Top with matcha powder and/or chia seeds if desired.

#166 Low-Carb with Kale

Replace spinach with kale or baby kale.

#167 Low-Carb with Chard

Replace spinach with Swiss chard.

#168 Spinach Apple Green Smoothie

302 Calories – 10g Carbs – 2.3g Fat – 7.9g Sugar – 9g Protein

Handful ice, 1 ripe banana, 1 green peeled green apple, 1 T ground flax seed, 1 C cold water, 2 Cs spinach.

Blend until frothy. Enjoy!

#169 Green Goddess Smoothie

327 Calories – 11g Carbs – 4.7g Fat – 15.9g Sugar – 9.4g Protein

2 T honey, 1 C almond milk, 2 t Matcha powder, ¼ cucumber, ½ mango, ½ bag frozen spinach, handful of fresh mint, 2 slices of melon of choice.

Blend everything until smooth.

#170 Green Goddess with Kale

Substitute spinach with kale or baby kale.

#171 Spinach Avocado Energy Smoothie

302 Calories – 9.9g Carbs – 10.5g Fat – 5.9g Sugar – 12.4g Protein

2 Cs water, 1 lemon, 1 t matcha green tea powder, 1 handful spinach, ½ banana, ½ avocado.

Blend until smooth.

#172 Kale Avocado Energy

Replace spinach with kale or baby kale.

#173 Spinach Pineapple Green Smoothie

318 Calories – 12.4g Carbs – 13g Fat – 7.9g Sugar – 13g Protein

¼-1/2 C apple juice, 1-2 handfuls ice, 1 C baby spinach, 1 C pineapple, 1 frozen banana, 2/3 C vanilla Greek yogurt.

Blend all components until well combined.

#174 Spinach Strawberry Green Smoothie

323 Calories – 12g Carbs – 8.9g Fat – 14.9g Sugar – 9g Protein

1 C ice, 1 C cold water, 3 Cs baby spinach, 2 mandarin oranges, 8-10 strawberries, 1.5 Cs frozen bananas.

Blend all ingredients until smooth in texture.

#175 Spinach and Cucumber Green Smoothie

218 Calories – 2.9g Carbs – 4g Fat – 15.2g Sugar – 12g Protein

1-2 Cs water, 1 scoop hemp protein powder, ½ green apple, ¾ C spinach, ½ cucumber.

Blend well until smooth.

#176 Spinach and Cucumber with Kiwi

Replace apple with 1 kiwi fruit.

#177 Ground Cherry Chutney

67 Calories – 15g Carbs – 1g Fat – 8g Sugar – 1g Protein

1 C ice, 1 C water, 1 t acai powder, 1 apple of choice, 1/3 C husked/ground cherries, 1-2 handfuls baby spinach.

Blend until well combined.

#178 Ground Cherry Chutney with Collard Greens

Replace spinach with collard greens or other veggie greens of choice.

#179 Spiced Apple Cider Smoothie

106 Calories – 19g Carbs – 3g Fat – 13g Sugar – 6g Protein

1 C water, 1 C ice, 1 T pumpkin seeds, 1 t cinnamon, 1 t nutmeg, 1 t ginger, ½ T apple cider vinegar, 1 chopped Fuji apple, 2 handfuls baby spinach. Blend ingredients until smooth in texture. Top with apple pieces and nuts.

#180 Thyme Traveler's Wife

51 Calories – 12g Carbs – 0g Fat – 9g Sugar – 1g Protein

Handful ice, 1 C coconut water, 2 sprigs thyme, ½ juiced lemon, ½ C frozen blueberries, 1-2 handfuls spinach.

Combine everything in a blender until you reach desired consistency. Top with a sprig of mint.

#181 Thyme Traveler's Wife with Kale

Replace spinach with kale or baby kale.

#182 Apple Zest Smoothie

77 Calories – 13g Carbs – 2g Fat – 8g Sugar – 2g Protein

1 C ice, 1 C water, ½ inch ginger, 1 T pumpkin seeds, ½ juiced lemon, 1 chopped apple of choice, 1 cucumber, 1-2 handfuls baby spinach.

Blend all components of smoothie until smooth. Top with extra pumpkin seeds.

#183 Apple Zest with Romaine

Replace spinach with romaine or baby romaine lettuce.

#184 Tropical Mojito Smoothie

104 Calories – 15g Carbs – 1g Fat – 13g Sugar – 1g Protein

½ C ice, 1 C water, 1 T flaxseed, ½ juiced lime, 8 mint leaves, 1 chopped green apple, ½ C frozen pineapple, 2 handfuls spinach.

Blend ingredients until smooth. Feel free to top with a sprig of mint.

#185 Lychee Ginger
120 Calories – 21g Carbs – 3g Fat – 17g Sugar – 4g Protein
½ C ice, 1 C water, 1 T hemp seed, ½ inch peeled ginger, ½ juiced lime, 6 peeled lychees, 1-2 handfuls spinach.
Incorporate ingredients together until combined.

#186 Lychee Ginger with Chard
Replace spinach with Swiss chard.

#187 Spinach, Avocado and Blueberry
201 Calories – 28g Carbs – 7g Fat – 3g Sugar – 5g Protein
1 scoop protein powder, ½ C crushed ice, 1 T honey, 1 T chia seeds, ½ ripe avocado, 1 C coconut milk, 1 C baby spinach, 1 C frozen blueberries.
Blend all ingredients until smooth.

#188 Refreshing Spinach Papaya Smoothie
189 Calories – 23g Carbs – 3g Fat – 14g Sugar – 3g Protein
Handful ice, 1 C coconut water, 1 juiced lime, 1 C baby spinach, ½ frozen banana, ½ ripe strawberry papaya with skin removed.
Pour in components of smoothie and blend until you reach consistency you like.

#189 Spinach Avocado Pineapple Smoothie
128 Calories – 18g Carbs – 1.9g Fat – 12.2g Sugar – 4.1g Protein
1 T chia seeds, 1 rip avocado, 1 C frozen pineapple chunks, 1 handful spinach.
Blend ingredients until combined thoroughly. Top with pineapple.

#190 "Popeye Went on a Vacation to Thailand" Smoothie
167 Calories – 13g Carbs – 2g Fat – 11g Sugar – 3g Protein
½ C coconut water, ½ C light coconut milk, 1 T fresh mint, 1 t freshly grated ginger, 1 C chopped frozen mango, 1 C spinach.
Pour all ingredients into your blender and combine on high until nice and smooth.

#191 Spinach Beet Happy Morning Smoothie

134 Calories – 9g Carbs – 2g Fat – 12.7g Sugar – 2g Protein

1 C ice, ½ C water, 2 Cs spinach, ½ orange, 1-2 handfuls frozen strawberries, 1 medium chopped beet.

Combine all ingredients until you achieve the consistency you desire. Enjoy this bright red drink right in the morning for a boost to your day! '

#192 Spinach and Grape Smoothie

150 Calories – 14g Carbs – 6g Fat – 11.4g Sugar – 3g Protein

1 T honey, 2 Cs ice cold water, 25 green seedless grapes, 2 handfuls baby spinach, 2 chopped apples of choice, 1 avocado.

Blend everything until smooth.

#193 Spinach Basil Smoothie

156 Calories – 19g Carbs – 2g Fat – 8.5g Sugar – 2g Protein

½ C crushed ice, 3 fresh basil leaves, ½ T honey , ½ C skim pr almond milk, ½ C plain Greek yogurt, 1 C spinach.

Blend ingredients until smooth and creamy.

#194 Savory Garden Green Smoothie

178 Calories – 13g Carbs – 0g Fat – 4g Sugar – 3.3g Protein

Few dashes Tabasco, sea salt (to taste), 1 C ice, few sprigs basil, ½ shallot, 2 small garlic cloves, ½ avocado, handful cherry tomatoes, handful orange bell pepper, handful yellow bell pepper, handful celery sticks, handful spinach leaves, 1 C ice cold filtered water.

Pour all ingredients in a blender, pulsing at first and then blending on high until you reach desired consistency. Enjoy this on-the-go liquid salad!

#195 Savory Green with Kale

Replace spinach with kale or baby kale.

#196 Savory Green with Chard

Substitute spinach with Swiss chard.

#197 Savory Green with Romaine

Replace spinach with romaine or baby romaine lettuce.

#198 Spinach Green Pepper Salad Smoothie

101.6 Calories – 19.6g Carbs – 10.3g Fat – 10.4g Sugar – 5.8g Protein

1 C water, 2 Cs raw spinach, 1 chopped green bell pepper, 3 stalks chopped celery, 1 chopped cucumber.

Combine ingredients until smooth.

#199 Non-Sweet Minty Green Smoothie

103 Calories – 12g Carbs – 2g Fat – 9.5g Sugar – 4g Protein

Handful mint, juice of ½ lemon or lime, 1-2 handfuls spinach or romaine, 2 stalks celery, 1/2 – 1 cucumber, 1 – 2 Cs water.

Blend until combined.

#200 Minty Green with Kale

Substitute spinach with kale or baby kale.

#201 Buttermilk Green Smoothie

123 Calories – 9g Carbs – 0.4g Fat – 4g Sugar – 2g Protein

1 T ground flax seed, small handful mint, 1 large handful spinach leaves, 1 chopped cucumber, 3 T plain Greek yogurt, ½ C buttermilk.

Blend all ingredients together until well combined and smooth.

#202 Buttermilk Green with Romaine

Replace spinach with romaine or baby romaine lettuce.

#203 Ranch House Salad Smoothie

133 Calories – 13g Carbs – 1g Fat – 5g Sugar – 2.6g Protein

Dashes of salt and pepper, 1 t dill, 1 t chives, 1 garlic clove, 1 C plain Greek yogurt, ½ onion, 2 carrots, 1 C spinach, 1 C romaine lettuce, ¼ avocado, 1 C water.

Incorporate ingredients together until smooth in texture.

#204 Ranch House Salad with Kale and Chard
Replace spinach and romaine lettuce with kale or baby kale and Swiss chard.

#205 Vegan Sweet Pea Smoothie
330 Calories – 26g Carbs – 11g Fat – 4g Sugar – 23g Protein
Handful ice, 8 drops stevia, ¼ t freshly grated ginger, ¼ t mint extract, ½ t almond extract, ¾ C almond milk, 1 handful fresh spinach, ½ avocado, 1 frozen banana, ½ C frozen peas, ½ C silken tofu.
Blend all components of smoothie recipe until combined and creamy in texture.

#206 Vegan Sweet Pea with Kale
Replace spinach with kale or baby kale.

#207 Vegan Sweet Pea with Collard Greens
Replace spinach with collard greens or other vegetable greens of choice, depending on the type of flavor you are aiming for.

Chapter 7: Broccoli Green Smoothies

#208 Broccoli Avocado Green Smoothie

178 Calories – 20g Carbs – 11g Fat – 9g Sugar – 3g Protein

1 C ice, 1 C vanilla almond milk, 1 T almond butter, 1 t matcha, ½ avocado, 1 chopped pear, 1.5 Cs broccoli florets.

Blend everything on high speed until well combined.

#209 Green Monster

89 Calories – 16g Carbs – 2g Fat – 10g Sugar – 3g Protein

1 C water, 1 C ice, 1 T hemp seed, 1 juiced lemon, 1 apple of choice, ½ C broccoli, 1 C cucumber.

Blend ingredients until you reach a smooth-like texture.

#210 Candied Carrot Tops with Broccoli

93 Calories – 15g Carbs – 0g Fat- 10g Sugar – 1g Protein

1 C ice, 1 C water, 1 piece candied ginger, ½ t camu powder, 1 C grapes of choice, 1 chopped carrot, 1 handful carrot greens, ½ C broccoli florets.

Blend components until smooth in texture.

#211 Apple Radish Mint Smoothie

135 Calories – 25 g Carbs – 1g Fat – 15g Sugar – 5g Protein

1 C ice, 1 C coconut water, 1 T flaxseed, 3 sprigs mint, 1 chopped baby radish, ½ C broccoli florets, 1 chopped Jon gold apple, 2 handfuls Mesclun.

Blend all ingredients together until you reach desired texture.

#212 Chamomile Lemonade Smoothie

75 Calories – 19g Carbs – 0g Fat – 14g Sugar – 1g Protein

1 C ice, ½ C water, 1 T matcha powder, 2 T chamomile flowers, ½ juiced lemon, ½ C grapes of choice, 1 peeled orange, 2 handfuls beet greens, ½ C broccoli florets.

Blend ingredients until combined well. Top with extra chamomile flowers.

#213 Purple Pineapple

158 Calories – 31g Carbs – 1g Fat – 18g Sugar – 7g Protein

1 C ice, 1 C water, 1 T flaxseed, 1 t maqui powder, ½ C frozen pineapple, 1 C grapes of choice, 1 purple cauliflower floret.

Blend until well combined. Smoothie will be a light-darkish purple color.

#214 The Swamp Smoothie
169 Calories – 30g Carbs – 2g Fat – 20g Sugar – 4g Protein
Stevia to taste, 1 T shelled hemp seeds, 3 T hemp protein powder, 1 T cacao powder, 1 C almond or hemp milk, 1 handful raw spinach, ½ C steamed but raw broccoli, ½ frozen banana, 1 C frozen strawberries.
Blend all ingredients until silky smooth. Enjoy this delectable smoothie any time of the day!

#215 Broccoli Banana Smoothie
184 Calories – 17g Carbs – 1g Fat – 2g Sugar – 2.9g Protein
1 T raw honey or maple syrup, 1 t ground cinnamon, 1 bunch of broccoli florets, 1 frozen banana, 1.5 Cs unsweetened almond milk.
Blend until smooth and creamy.

#216 Blueberry Broccoli Smoothie
143 Calories – 12g Carbs – 0.4g Fat – 1g Sugar – 4g Protein
½ C raisins, 2 T sunflower seeds, 1 C oats, 1 C broccoli, 1 frozen banana, 1 C frozen blueberries, 1 C dairy free milk, 1 C water.
Combine everything until you reach a smooth texture you desire.

#217 Refreshing Raw Broccoli Smoothie
109 Calories – 10g Carbs – 0g Fat – 1.5g Sugar – 3g Protein
1 C ice, 2 T mashed avocado, 1 T fresh lemon juice, 1 frozen banana, ½ C raw broccoli, ¾ C apple juice.
Blend until combined.

#218 Pineapple Broccoli Green Smoothie
339 Calories – 74g Carbs – 13g Fat- 7g Sugar – 9g Protein
1 C unsweetened almond milk, 1-2 Cs baby spinach, 1 frozen banana, 1.5 Cs frozen pineapple chunks, 1 C frozen broccoli.
Blend ingredients together until smooth and frothy in texture. Top with almonds.

#219 Broccoli Banana Peanut Butter Green Smoothie

172 Calories – 32g Carbs – 9g Fat – 11g Sugar – 5g Protein

1 C ice cold water, ½ C baby spinach, ½ T peanut butter, 1 C frozen broccoli, 1 frozen banana.

Combine ingredients until creamy.

#220 Basic Banana and Broccoli Smoothie

152 Calories – 37g Carbs – 10g Fat – 7g Sugar – 4g Protein

1 C ice cold water, 2 Cs frozen broccoli, 2 frozen bananas.

Blend until smooth in texture.

#221 Broccoli Grapefuit Detox Smoothie

264 Calories – 55g Carbs – 9g Fat – 11g Sugar – 7g Protein

1 C unsweetened almond milk, ½ red grapefruit, and 1 C fresh or frozen broccoli, 1 frozen banana.

Combine until you reach desired consistency.

#222 Broccoli Sprout Smoothie

230 Calories – 23g Carbs – 17g Fat – 9g Sugar – 16g Protein

4 dates, ½ t vanilla extract, 1 t carob powder, 1 T cacao powder, 1 T maca powder, 2 T flax seed meal, 1 C frozen pineapple chunks, 1 C frozen strawberries, 1 frozen banana, 2 C broccoli sprouts, 2 Cs baby spinach, 1.2 C raw almonds, 3 Cs ice cold water.

Blend all ingredients together until you form a nice, cream green smoothie.

#223 Super Green and Creamy Smoothie

180 Calories – 23g Carbs – 13g Fat – 7g Sugar – 12g Protein

Handful ice, handful baby spinach leaves, ½ C broccoli florets, 1 Swiss chard, 1 frozen banana, 1 C coconut water.

Blend ingredients together until thoroughly combined.

#224 Delicious Morning Smoothie

450 Calories – 22g Carbs – 38g Fat – 18g Sugar – 59g Protein

1 scoop green powder, 1 T spirulina powder, 1 t ground turmeric, 1 t ground cinnamon, 1 t pure vanilla extract, 2 dates, 2 T natural sweetener of choice, ½ chopped apple of choice, ½ frozen banana, 1 scoop protein powder of choice, ½ C vanilla almond milk, handful broccoli, handful spinach, handful lettuce, handful baby kale, handful chard, handful arugula, 2 T almond butter, ½ avocado, 1 C frozen blueberries.

Combine everything on high speed until combined. This may take a few minutes due to amount of smoothie components. A very filling smoothie to consume in the morning!

#225 Fruit and Veggie Green Smoothie

70 Calories – 6g Carbs – 0g Fat – 2g Sugar – 4g Protein

1 C grapefruit juice, 1 carrot, 1 orange, ¼ apple of choice, 1 handful spinach leaves, 1 handful broccoli florets.

Blend ingredients until creamy.

#226 Creamy Spring Green Strawberry Smoothie

159 Calories – 14g Carbs – 3g Fat – 9g Sugar – 3.5g Protein

1 C unsweetened almond milk, 1 head of broccoli, ½ avocado, 1 handful spinach, 8-10 frozen strawberries.

Blend until creamy.

#227 Everything Smoothie

150 Calories – 28g Carbs – 12g Fat – 2g Sugar – 8g Protein

1 C ice, ¼ frozen banana, 1 C frozen strawberries, ½ C spinach, ½ C frozen broccoli, 1 C chopped carrots, ½ C frozen pineapple chunks, ½ C frozen peach slices, 1 peeled orange, ½ C red or green grapes, ½ C soy milk.

Blend everything until you reach a creamy consistency. A great way to get many food groups in!

#228 5 A Day Smoothie
340 Calories – 16g Carbs – 12g Fat – 7g Sugar – 16g Protein
1 C coconut water, 1.5 Cs apple juice, ½ inch ginger root, 1 avocado, 2 broccoli florets, 1 handful spinach leaves, 2 handfuls kale, 2 handfuls frozen peas.
Blend until creamy.

#229 Healthy Broccoli Smoothie
140 Calories – 11g Carbs – 2g Fat – 1.9g Sugar – 8g Protein
1 C orange juice, 2 mandarin oranges, 2 Cs spinach leaves, 4 broccoli florets, 1 C chopped carrot.
Combine in blender until smooth.

#230 Monster Smoothie
290 Calories – 24g Carbs – 7g Fat – 11g Sugar – 10g Protein
1 C apple-strawberry juice, 1 frozen banana, 1 C frozen strawberries, ½ C spinach, ½ C broccoli.
Blend until creamy. Serve with strawberry slices as garnish.

#231 Red Smoothie Bowl
369 Calories – 37g Carbs – 10g Fat – 17g Sugar – 11g Protein
2 T coconut cream, handful ice, ½ C coconut water, 2 t flax seed meal, ½ celery stalk, 1 beet, 4 frozen strawberries, 2 broccoli florets, 1 handful spinach, ½ C cucumber, ½ C frozen mango, 1 frozen banana.
Blend until creamy. Pour in a bowl and garnish with fruit and mint leaves.

Chapter 8: Packing the Protein

#232 Berry Protein Smoothie
318 Calories – 21.2g Carbs – 14.6g Fat – 23.6g Sugars – 34.7g Protein
1 C frozen spinach, ½ frozen banana, ½ C frozen mixed berries, 1 scoop vanilla protein powder, 1 C water.
Pour all ingredients in blend and mix until smooth.

#233 Berry Protein with Kale
Substitute spinach with kale or baby kale.

#234 Berry Protein with Romaine
Replace spinach with romaine or baby romaine lettuce.

#235 Citrus Protein Green Smoothie
339 Calories – 19.5g Carbs – 3.4g Fat – 29.3g Sugar – 40.2g Protein
1 T honey, 2 Cs frozen spinach, 1 C strawberries, 1 frozen banana, 1 orange, ½ large grapefruit, 2 T vanilla protein powder, 1.5 Cs unsweetened vanilla almond milk.
Pour all ingredients in a blender and combine on high speed until creamy.

#236 Apple Breeze Protein Green Smoothie
317 Calories – 7.5g Carbs – 4.4g Fat – 11g Sugar – 20.1g Protein
½ C water, ½ C frozen raspberries, ½ C organic apple juice, 1 scoop of protein powder, ½ C spinach.
Blend until smooth.

#237 Citrus Berry Protein Green Smoothie
302 Calories – 6.7g Carbs – 5g Fat – 9g Sugar – 20.1g Protein
½ C 100% orange juice, 1 C frozen strawberries, 1 C water, 1 scoop protein powder, ½ C spinach.
Blend until combined.

#238 Strawberry Lemonade Protein Green Smoothie
312 Calories – 8.3g Carbs – 5g Fat – 6.9g Sugar – 20.1g Protein
Freshly squeezed lemon juice, 1 C frozen strawberries, 1 C water, 1 C spinach, 1 scoop protein powder.
Combine until thoroughly mixed. Top with strawberry slices.

#239 Strawberry Peach Paradise Protein Smoothie
307 Calories – 7.4g Carbs – 4.5g Fat – 9g Sugar – 20.2g Protein
½ C frozen strawberries, ½ C frozen peaches, 1 C water, 1 scoop protein powder, ½ C spinach.
Blend until combined. Enjoy ice cold.

#240 Green Berry Blues Protein Smoothie

319 Calories – 9g Carbs – 4.9g Fat – 8.4g Sugar – 20.2g Protein

1 C frozen blueberries, 1 C almond milk, 1 scoop protein powder, 1/2-1 C spinach. Blend until smooth.

#241 Green-Berry Blues with Kale

Replace spinach with kale or baby kale.

#242 Green-Berry Blue with Collard Greens

Replace spinach with collard greens or other veggie greens of choice, depending on what flavor you are aiming for.

#243 Peanut Butter Banana Protein Smoothie

324 Calories – 12.4g Carbs – 9g Fat – 10.4g Sugar – 20.2g Protein

¼ C water, ¾ C almond milk, 1-2 t natural peanut butter, 1 frozen banana, 1 scoop protein powder, ½ C spinach.

Combine in blender until smooth and creamy.

#244 Citrus Berry Protein Smoothie

317 Calories – 11.9g Carbs – 10g Fat – 11.7g Sugar – 20g Protein

½ C 100% orange juice, ½ C frozen strawberries, 1 C water, 1 scoop protein powder, 1 C spinach.

Blend until thoroughly combined.

#245 Triple Green Protein Smoothie

144 Calories – 20.6g Carbs – 0.8g Fat – 13.2g Sugar – 15.3g Protein

Sweetener of choice, to taste, 1-2 handfuls ice, 1 C kale, 1 C spinach, 1-2 T water, ½ C plain Greek yogurt, ½ C honeydew.

Blend until creamy, adding sweetener if needed to truly satisfy taste buds. Enjoy!

#246 Savory Green Protein Smoothie

108 Calories – 17g Carbs – 1.8g Fat – 6g Sugar – 32g Protein

½ - 1 C ice, 2 pinches red pepper, 2 pinches salt, ½ t Tony Chachere's seasoning, 5-7 basil leaves, 1 stalk rosemary, 2/3 C unsweetened plain almond milk, 1 C plain Greek yogurt, 3 Cs raw spinach, 2-3 whole heirloom tomatoes.

Blend ingredients together until smooth and slightly frothy.

#247 Savory Green with Kale
Replace spinach with kale or baby kale.

#248 Savory Green with Chard
Replace spinach with Swiss chard.

#249 Vanilla Green Protein Smoothie
182 Calories – 20g Carbs – 3g Fat – 8g Sugar – 18g Protein
½ C ice, 1 scoop vanilla protein powder, 1 C fresh baby spinach, 1 C unsweetened almond milk, 1 frozen/ripe banana.
Blend until creamy and frothy on top.

#250 Vanilla Green with Romaine
Replace spinach with romaine or baby romaine lettuce.

#251 Green Warrior Protein Smoothie
209 Calories – 14g Carbs – 0g Fat – 4g Sugar – 17g Protein
Handful ice, 1.5 t virgin coconut oil, 2 T fresh mint leaves, 1/3 C frozen mango, 3-4 T hemp hearts, 1 stalk celery, 1 C chopped cucumber, 1 chopped apple of choice, 1 C baby spinach, ½ C red grapefruit juice.
Blend until creamy and thoroughly combined. Enjoy!

#252 Green Warrior with Kale
Replace spinach with kale or baby kale.

#253 Green Warrior with Collard Greens
Replace spinach with collard greens or other veggie greens of choice, depending on what kind of flavor you are trying to achieve.

#254 Very Berry Super Smoothie
480 Calories – 54g Carbs – 11g Fat – 9g Sugar – 58g Protein
1 T ground flaxseed, 1 T walnuts, 2 scoops vanilla protein powder, ½ C plain Greek yogurt, 2 Cs frozen mixed berries, 1 C spinach, and 1.5 Cs water.
Blend until creamy. Garnish with additional frozen berries if you choose.

#255 Apple and Great Grains Smoothie

435 Calories – 46g Carbs – 13g Fat – 9g Sugar – 59g Protein

Couple dashes of cinnamon, handful ice, ¼ C uncooked oats, 2 T almonds, 1 C spinach, 1 chopped apple of choice, 2 scoops vanilla protein powder, 1.5 Cs of almond milk.

Combine ingredients until silky smooth. Sprinkle cinnamon over top and serve.

#256 Apple and Great Grains with Romaine

Replace spinach with romaine or baby romaine lettuce.

#257 Chocolate, Peanut Butter and Banana Protein Smoothie

485 Calories – 38g Carbs – 22g Fat – 8g Sugar – 59g Protein

1 T cacao nibs or dark cocoa powder, 2 T natural peanut butter, 1 C spinach, 1 frozen banana, 2 scoops chocolate protein powder, 1.5 Cs almond milk or plain Greek yogurt.

Mix components of smoothie together in a blender on high speed until smooth. Garnish with additional cacao nibs or powder.

#258 Chocolate, PB and Banana with Kale

Substitute spinach for kale or baby kale.

#259 Strawberry Banana Protein Smoothie

490 Calories – 47g Carbs – 9g Fat – 11g Sugar – 55g Protein

2 T ground flax seed, 1 C spinach, 1 C frozen strawberries, 1 frozen banana, 2 scoop vanilla or strawberry flavored protein powder, 1.5 Cs almond milk or plain Greek yogurt.

Blend ingredients until thoroughly combined and silky smooth. Top with strawberry slices.

#260 Strawberry Banana with Kale

Replace spinach with kale or baby kale.

#261 Strawberry Banana with Chard

Replace spinach with Swiss chard.

#262 Chocolate Cherry Awesomeness Protein Smoothie

430 Calories – 47g Carbs – 13g Fat – 9g Sugar – 56g Protein

1 T cacao nibs or dark cocoa powder, 1 T ground flax seed, 1 T walnuts, 1 C spinach, 2 Cs sweet dark cherries, 1 scoops chocolate protein powder, 1.5 Cs chocolate almond milk.

Combine until smooth and garnish with additional walnuts and a cherry.

#263 Vanilla Pumpkin Pie Protein Smoothie

490 Calories – 45g Carbs – 13g Fat – 13g Sugar – 69g Protein

Handful ice, cinnamon and vanilla extract (to taste), 1 T ground flax seed, 1 T walnuts, ¾ C pureed pumpkin, 2 scoops vanilla protein powder, 1.5 Cs almond milk of plain Greek yogurt, ½ C kale.

Combine smoothie components until silky smooth. Garnish with dash of cinnamon and additional walnuts. Enjoy!

#264 Vanilla Pumpkin Pie with Spinach

Replace Kale with spinach or baby spinach leaves.

#265 Baked Apple Protein Smoothie

491 Calories – 36g Carbs – 15g Fat – 10g Sugar – 57g Protein

Handful ice, cinnamon (to taste), 1 T sesame seeds, 1 T ground flax seed, 1 T almonds, 1 C spinach, 1 chopped appleof choice, 2 scoops vanilla protein powder, 1.5 Cs almond milk or plain Greek yogurt.

Blend everything well until creamy. Top with cinnamon and additional almonds.

#266 Baked Apple with Kale

Replace spinach with kale or baby kale.

#267 Tropical Power Protein Smoothie

495 Calories – 46g Carbs – 12g Fat – 8.5g Sugar – 58g Protein

½ C plain Greek yogurt, 2 T unsweetened coconut flakes, 1 T ground flax seed, 1 C spinach, 1 C frozen pineapple, ½ frozen banana, 2 scoops vanilla protein powder, 1.5 Cs almond milk or water.

Blend until thoroughly combined. Top with additional coconut flakes if desired.

#268 Super Food Smoothie
329 Calories – 52g Carbs – 4g Fat – 11g Sugar – 28g Protein
1 T ground flax seed, 1 scoop chocolate protein powder, ½ C frozen blueberries, ½ frozen banana, ½ C frozen strawberries, ½ C chopped raw beets, 1 C water, ½ C frozen cherries, 1 C spinach.
Blend all ingredients on high until combined and creamy. Garnish with a cherry.

#269 Super Food with Kale
Replace spinach with kale or baby kale.

#270 Super Food with Chard
Replace spinach with Swiss chard.

#271 Dr. Mike's Power Smoothie
389 Calories – 34g Carbs – 17g Fat – 11g Sugar – 33g Protein
Handful ice, 1.5 Cs water, 2 T chopped walnuts, 2 T flax seed meal, 1 scoop vanilla protein powder, 1 C frozen or fresh blueberries, ¼ C low far cottage cheese, ½ C spinach.
Combine until creamy and smooth. Top with additional chopped walnuts.

#272 Double Chocolate Mint Protein Smoothie
292 Calories – 32g Carbs – 12g Fat – 8.5g Sugar – 25g Protein
¼ C water, handful ice, 2 mint leaves, 1 T cacao nibs, 2 T cocoa powder, 1 T walnuts, ¾ C dark chocolate almond milk, 1 scoop chocolate protein powder, 1 C spinach.
Blend all ingredients together on high speed until you reach a smooth, silky consistency. Top with mint leaf and additional cacao nibs.

#273 Double Chocolate Mint with Collard Greens
Replace spinach with collard greens or other vegetable greens of choice, depending on what kind of flavor you want to achieve.

#274 Coconut Almond Protein Smoothie
405 Calories – 33g Carbs – 21g Fat – 12g Sugar – 27g Protein
Handful ice, 1.5 Cs water, 1 T almond butter, 1 C dark chocolate almond milk, 1 T unsweetened coconut flakes, 1 scoop chocolate protein powder, 1 C spinach.
Combine components until you reach desired texture. Garnish with additional coconut.

#275 Coconut Almond with Kale
Replace spinach with kale or baby kale.

#276 Blueberry Breakfast Protein Smoothie
436 Calories – 59g Carbs – 18g Fat – 12g Sugar – 42g Protein
1 T chia seeds, 2 T oats, 2 T walnuts, 1.5 scoops protein powder, ½ frozen banana, 1 C frozen blueberries, ½ C kale.
Blend until smooth. Top with additional berries.

#277 Blueberry Breakfast with Spinach
Replace kale with spinach or baby spinach.

#278 Mango Tango Protein Smoothie
469 Calories – 74g Carbs – 20g Fat – 14g Sugar – 53g Protein
Handful ice, 1.5 Cs orange juice, 1 T walnuts, 1 C chopped frozen mango chunks, 2 scoops vanilla protein powder, 1 C spinach.
Blend until combined and silky. Top with additional chopped walnuts if desired.

#279 The Green Protein Monster
346 Calories – 62g Carbs – 12g Fat – 11g Sugar – 9g Protein
Handful ice, ½ avocado, 1 strip of a lemon rind, ½ C frozen mango chunks, 1 C grapes of choice, 2 stalks kale, 1-1.5 Cs water.
Combine ingredients until smooth and creamy. Top with lemon wedge.

#280 Green Protein Monster with Spinach
Substitute kale with spinach or baby spinach.

Chapter 9: Totes to Oats

#281 Green Power Oat Smoothie

110 Calories – 22g Carbs – 3g Fat – 13g Sugar – 2g Protein

1 C ice, 1 t lemon juice, 1 T honey, ½ C chopped green apple, ¼ C parsley leaves, 1 C baby spinach, ¾ C unsweetened coconut milk, ¼ C quick oats.

Incorporate all ingredients together until well combined and smooth.

#282 Green Power with Kale

Replace spinach with kale or baby kale.

#283 Oat, Blueberry and Banana Smoothie

154 Calories – 24g Carbs – 4g Fat – 15.5g Sugar – 3g Protein

1 C ice, 3 Cs baby spinach, 1.5 Cs frozen blueberries, 1 frozen banana, ½ C vanilla Greek yogurt, ¼ C whole grain oats, 1 C orange juice.

Blend ingredients until smooth in texture.

#284 Lean Green Oat Breakfast Smoothie

123 Calories – 29g Carbs – 5.9g Fat – 18g Sugar – 5g Protein

1 T chia seeds, ½ C whole rolled oats, ¾ C plain Greek yogurt, ¾ C orange juice, 1 frozen banana, ½ C frozen blueberries, 2 Cs spinach.

Blend all ingredients until nice and silky smooth. Top with extra chia seeds.

#285 Pear and Oat Green Smoothie

116 Calories – 21g Carbs – 9g Fat – 12g Sugar – 24.5g Protein

1 t super boost powder, 2-3 Cs water, ½ C oats, 1 scoop protein powder of choice, 1 frozen banana, half a pear, 1 C spinach, ½ cucumber.

Mix components together to make a boosting breakfast or mid-day smoothie!

#286 Oat, Kale and Blueberry Smoothie

121 Calories – 17g Carbs – 8g Fat – 12.5g Sugar – 5.5g Protein

Handful ice, 1 t honey, ¼ C almond milk, ½ frozen banana, 3 T raw oats, 2 T Greek yogurt, ½ C frozen blueberries, ½ C kale leaves. Optional: flaxseed, vanilla extract and cinnamon.

Blend all ingredients together until smooth. Sprinkle with cinnamon if desired.

#287 Green Power Oat Smoothie

146 Calories – 25g Carbs – 10g Fat – 11g Sugar – 6g Protein

½ C ice, 1 t lemon juice, 1 T honey, ½ chopped green apple, ¼ C parsley leaves, 1 C baby spinach, ¾ C unsweetened coconut milk, ¼ C quick or old fashioned oats. Blend components together until you reach desired consistency.

#288 A Kale Oatmeal Smoothie

119 Calories – 18g Carbs – 8g Fat – 12.5g Sugar – 5g Protein

1 C almond milk, handful ice, honey to taste, 1 T chia seeds of flaxseed meal, 1 T natural peanut or almond butter, 1 C baby kale, 1 frozen banana, ½ C old-fashioned rolled oats.
Blend everything until silky smooth.

#289 Oat Spinach Banana Smoothie

128 Calories – 21g Carbs – 11g Fat – 11g Sugar – 4.5g Protein

3-4 Cs raw spinach, 1 T honey, 1 C low-fat or soy milk, ½ C raw oats, 1 frozen banana.
Blend until completely combined. Top with banana slices if you choose.

#290 Green Morning Smoothie

165 Calories – 35g Carbs – 2g Fat – 20g Sugar – 3g Protein

2 frozen bananas, 1 t vanilla extract, 1 T honey, 1 C baby spinach, 1 C ice, 1.25 Cs frozen mango chunks, ½ C whole oats, and 2 Cs vanilla almond milk.
Incorporate all ingredients until mixture is smooth in texture. A tasty breakfast treat!

#291 Berry Spinach Oatmeal Smoothie

145 Calories – 28g Carbs – 3g Fat – 18g Sugar – 2.5g Protein

½ C frozen mixed berries, ¾ C low fat or soy milk, ¼ C old fashioned oats, 1 T ground flaxseed, ¾ C plain Greek yogurt, ½ C baby spinach.
Blend until combined.

#292 Mango Spinach Oatmeal Smoothie

169 Calories – 38g Carbs – 4g Fat – 23g Sugar – 2g Protein

½ C ice, ¼ C Greek yogurt, ¼ C whole oatmeal, ½ C baby spinach, 1 C chopped mango, 2 Cs almond milk.

Mix components together to create a silky smooth texture.

#293 Blueberry Spinach Breakfast Smoothie

134 Calories – 24g Carbs – 5g Fat – 16g Sugar – 1g Protein

1/8 t cinnamon, ¾ C almond milk, ½ C plain Greek yogurt, 1 C frozen banana, 1 C frozen or fresh spinach, 3 T old fashioned oats.

Blend oats for about 30 seconds before pouring in remaining ingredients. Pulse/blend until smooth. Garnish with additional blueberries.

#294 Strawberry Banana Oatmeal Smoothie

161 Calories – 21g Carbs – 2g Fat – 14g Sugar – 21g Protein

¼ C old fashioned rolled oats, 1 C frozen strawberries, ½ frozen banana, 1 C baby spinach, 1 scoop protein powder of choice, ½ C pomegranate juice, ½ C unsweetened almond milk.

Blend ingredients until smoothie mixture is completely smooth.

#295 Ruby Red Oats Smoothie

191 Calories – 26g Carbs – 2.3g Fat – 13.4g Sugar – 20.5g Protein

1-2 handfuls ice, ½ frozen banana, 1/3 C frozen raspberries, 4-5 frozen strawberries, 1 roasted/peeled beet, 2/3 Cs water, ½ C pomegranate juice, 1/3 C plain Greek yogurt, 1 scoop vanilla protein powder, 1 t chia seeds, 1 t flax seed, 1/3 C old fashioned oats.

Blend all ingredients until smooth in texture. This may take a few minutes. Will be a nice ruby red color when completed! Enjoy!

#296 Peaches and Cream Oatmeal Smoothie

331 Calories – 46g Carbs – 4g Fat – 12g Sugar – 29g Protein

1 C almond milk, ¼ t vanilla extract, ¼ C oatmeal, 1 C plain Greek yogurt, 1 C frozen peach slices 1 handful spinach leaves.

Blend everything until smooth.

#297 Banana Oatmeal Breakfast Smoothie

279 Calories – 49g Carbs – 3g Fat – 11g Sugar – 17g Protein

¼ t ground cinnamon, 1 t honey, ½ C almond milk, 1 frozen banana, ½ C plain Greek yogurt, ¼ C old fashioned rolled oats, 1 C kale.

Combine ingredients until creamy and top with sprinkle of cinnamon.

#298 Chocolate Banana Green Smoothie

268 Calories – 46g Carbs – 8g Fat – 12.3g Sugar – 29g Protein

1 T cocoa powder, 1 C plain Greek yogurt, 1 C almond milk, 10 almonds, 1 frozen banana, 1 t coconut flakes, 1 t peanut butter, 1 C kale or spinach.

Blend until smooth and creamy. Garnish with additional coconut.

#299 Hearty Fruit n' Oat Green Smoothie

235 Calories – 34g Carbs – 8.5g Fat – 11g Sugar – 9g Protein

1 t maple syrup, ½ C old fashioned oats, ¼ C raw almonds, 1 frozen banana, 1 C frozen strawberries, 1 C vanilla Greek yogurt, 1 C spinach.

Chapter 10: Caffeine for your Green

#300 Banana Berry Green Tea Smoothie

210 Calories – 12.2g Carbs – 1.9g Fat – 19.5g Sugar – 3.5g Protein

1-2 handfuls ice, ½ frozen banana, 1.5 T raw honey, 1 C frozen mixed berries, 6 bags brewed green tea, ½ C spinach.

Prepare green tea, blend the ingredients and mix until combine. Drink chilled!

#301 Banana Berry Green with Chard

Replace spinach with Swiss chard.

#302 Avocado Matcha Smoothie

259 Calories – 11g Carbs – 4.5g Fat – 9.9g Sugar – 6.7g Protein

2 T hemp seed, 1 t Matcha powder, 1 C almond milk, ½ avocado, 2 Cs spinach. Blend until combine.

#303 Mango Green Tea Smoothie

299 Calories – 13g Carbs – 8g Fat – 15.4g Sugar – 10g Protein

1 handful mint, 1 T fresh lemon juice, 2 Cs spinach, 2 ripe bananas, 1.5 Cs frozen mango, 1.5 Cs brewed and chill green tea of choice.

Blend all components together until well combined. Garnish with mint leaf.

#304 Mango Green Tea with Kale

Replace spinach with kale or baby kale.

#305 Vanilla Matcha Green Tea Latte Smoothie

320 Calories – 9g Carbs – 3.4g Fat – 13.9g Sugar – 4.8g Protein

1 T honey, ½ C vanilla almond milk, ½ C hot water, ½ t matcha powder, ½ C spinach. Blend until combined. Top with sugar free whipped cream if desired.

#306 Green Tea Nectarine Smoothie

51 Calories – 12g Carbs – 0g Fat – 9g Sugar – 1g Protein

1 C ice, 1 C water, 1 t matcha powder, 1 pitted nectarine, ½ C grapes, 1.5 Cs chard. Blend until smooth.

#307 The Macarena

211 Calories – 24g Carbs – 12g Fat – 12g Sugar – 5g Protein

1 C water, 1 T chia seeds, 1/8 t nutmeg, 3 brazil nuts, ½ t maca powder, ½ t matcha powder, 1 nectarine, 1 pear, 2 handfuls red leaf lettuce.
Blend until combined and silky.

#308 Earl Grey Green Tea Smoothie

73 Calories – 15g Carbs – 2g Fat – 9g Sugar – 1g Protein

1 C ice, 1 C water, 1 T flaxseed, 1.5 T earl grey tea, 1 pear, ¼ C frozen blueberries, 1-2 handfuls mixed lettuce.
Blend until well combined. For a stronger tea flavor, add in steeped tea leaves and blend as well.

#309 Mint Green Tea Smoothie

163 Calories – 40g Carbs – 0g Fat – 29g Sugar – 2g Protein

1 C ice, ½ C water, 10 mint leaves, ½ t matcha powder, 1 C grapes of choice, 1 peeled orange, 1-2 handfuls chard.
Blend until thick in texture. Feel free to add more water to reach desired consistency.

#310 Hibiscus Tea Smoothie

123 Calories – 19g Carbs – 5g Fat – 13g Sugar – 3g Protein

½ C ice, 1 C water, 2 T raw almonds, 1 chopped pear, ½ C frozen strawberries, 2 T dried hibiscus, 1 C boy choy.
Blend ingredients together until you have a pink in color smoothie mixture.

#311 Goji Green Tea Smoothie

153 Calories – 21g Carbs – 6g Fat – 13g Sugar – 5g Protein

½ C ice, 1 C water, 1 T matcha powder, 1 T goji berries, ¼ C raw cashews, 1 chopped green apple, 1-2 handfuls spinach.
Incorporate ingredients together until thoroughly combined.

#312 Sweet Potato Energy Smoothie

102 Calories – 13.7g Carbs – 8.1g Fat – 4g Sugar – 26g Protein

1 t vanilla, ½-1 t cinnamon, 2 t instant espresso powder, 1 scoop protein powder of your choosing, 1.5 Cs almond milk, 1 C frozen sweet potato.
Blend everything together until silky smooth. Top with additional cinnamon.

#313 Green Tea Smoothie

164 Calories – 36g Carbs – 0g Fat – 22g Sugar – 8g Protein

½ C ice, ½ C baby spinach, 1 t honey, ¼ C plain Greek yogurt, 1 frozen banana, ¾ C brewed and chilled green tea.

Blend ingredients together until smooth.

#314 Chocolate Mocha Protein Smoothie

390 Calories – 45g Carbs – 18g Fat – 12g Sugar – 67g Protein

1 t cacao nibs, 1 t unsweetened shredded/dried coconut, 1 handful spinach, 1 C frozen broccoli, ½ frozen banana, ¼ t cinnamon, 1 T cocoa powder, 1.5 scoops mocha protein powder, 2 C almonds.

Combine components until thoroughly mixed.

#315 Ginger Peach Green Tea Smoothie

127 Calories – 23g Carbs – 12g Fat – 9g Sugar – 3g Protein

½ t freshly grated ginger, ½ frozen banana, ½ C vanilla Greek yogurt, 1 C frozen sliced peaches, ½ C brewed green tea of choice.

Blend all ingredients together until you reach a smooth yet frothy texture.

#316 Bulletproof Banana Green Smoothie

243 Calories – 31g Carbs – 15g Fat – 12g Sugar – 19g Protein

Handful ice, 1-2 pinches cayenne pepper, 2 cloves garlic, 1 t salt, 1 avocado, 1 chopped cucumber, 1 C chopped carrot, 1 C coconut water, 1 T almond butter, 1-2 T coconut butter, 1 frozen banana, ½ scoop vanilla protein powder, ½ C spinach, 1 C brewed black coffee of choice.

Blend all ingredients on high until you reach your desired consistency.

Chapter 11: Rich in Green Fruit-Free

#317 Spring Detox Smoothie

187 Calories – 2.3g Carbs – 3g Fat – 2.9g Sugar – 10.2g Protein

1-2 handfuls ice, 2 T freshly squeezed lemon juice, 1 C coconut water, ½ C micro greens and/or pea shoots, ½ C raw arugula, 1 C raw kale, ½ avocado, ½ cucumber. Blend all components together, pulsing until well combined. Scrape sides of blender if needed.

#318 Fruit-Free Green Smoothie

175 Calories – 3g Carbs – 4.3g Fat – 1.8g Sugar – 9.3g Protein

1-2 handfuls ice, 1 C coconut water, 2 Cs raw spinach, ½ avocado, ½ peeled lemon, ¼ C parsley, ½ cucumber.
Blend ingredients until smooth.

#319 Drinkable Salad Smoothie

75 Calories – 3.4g Carbs – 1g Fat – 2.9g Sugar – 11g Protein

Salt, dill and chive to taste, 1 t pumpkin seed oil, 2 t fresh parsley, 1 C vanilla Greek yogurt, 1 seeded jalapeño pepper, 1 handful lettuce, 1 chopped cucumber.
Incorporate ingredients until completely combined and smooth.

#320 No-Fruit Pumpkin Green Smoothie

116 Calories – 4g Carbs – 2.3g Fat – 4g Sugar – 3.9g Protein

Handful of ice, pinch of nutmeg, ½ inch piece of ginger, ¼ t pumpkin pie spice, ¼ t ground cinnamon, ¼ C raw cashews, ½ C coconut water, ¾ C pumpkin puree, 1 C fresh kale.
Blend all ingredients on high until thick and smooth in texture.

#321 No-Fruit Creamy Green Smoothie

98 Calories – 2g Carbs – 1g Fat – 2g Sugar – 1.5g Protein

2 t raspberry-lemon magnesium supplement, 1 T hemp seeds or hemp hearts, 1/3 C raw cashews, ¾ C water, 1 C ice, 2 Cs kale.
Blend ingredients until combined to desired consistency.

#322 Creamy No-Fruit Allowed Smoothie
56 Calories – 2g Carbs – 0g Fat – 1g Sugar – 1g Protein
1 C ice, pinch sea salt, 1 t vanilla extract, 1 C oats, 3 Cs water, 1/3 C coconut butter, 2 C spinach.
Combine everything until well blended and creamy.

#323 Fruit-Free Monster Protein Smoothie
98 Calories – 12g Carbs – 1g Fat – 2g Sugar – 29g Protein
½ large avocado, 1 scoop berry blast flavored protein powder, 1 C unsweetened almond milk, 2 handfuls baby spinach.
Blend until frothy.

#324 Healthy Thin Mint Smoothie
159 Calories – 20g Carbs – 4g Fat – 3g Sugar – 2g Protein
2 Cs ice, 1 T maple syrup. 1 C baby spinach, ¼ C dark chocolate chips, 1 C almond milk, ¼ C fresh mint, ¾ C plain Greek yogurt.
Combine until it reaches consistency that you desire.

Chapter 12: Kick it Up a Notch

#325 Cinnamon Apple Green Smoothie

289 Calories – 13.3g Carbs – 6.2g Fat – 12.9g Sugar – 12.9g Protein

1 T cinnamon, ¼ C almonds, ½ C Greek yogurt, ½ C almond milk, ½ apple of choice, 2 Cs spinach.

Blend everything until silky smooth. Top with a pinch of cinnamon.

#326 Zucchini Bread Smoothie

225 Calories – 32g Carbs – 12g Fat – 15g Sugar – 5g Protein

1 C ice, 1 C vanilla almond milk, ¼ C walnuts, ½ t cinnamon, 1 t mesquite powder, 1 chopped pear, 1 chopped zucchini, 1-2 Cs boy choy.

Combine all ingredients until smooth in texture. Top with extra walnuts.

#327 Spicy Vegetable Smoothie

39 Calories – 9g Carbs – 0g Fat – 4g Sugar – 1g Protein

½ C ice, 1 C water, 4 sprigs cilantro, ½ seeded jalapeño, ½ juiced lime, 2 stalks celery, 1 cucumber, 2 heirloom tomatoes, 1-2 handfuls spinach.

Pulse frequently until all components are quite small, and then blend until smooth.

#328 Cinnamon Spice Butternut Squash Parfait

143 Calories – 12.3g Carbs – 8.1g Fat – 13g Sugar – 4g Protein

½ t nutmeg, 1 t vanilla, 1 t cinnamon, 2 T hemp hearts, 3 T maple syrup, 1.5 Cs roasted buttermilk squash, 1 C plant milk.

Roast squash after de-seeding for 30 minutes in a 350 degree preheated over. Allow to cool, and then toss in blender with remaining ingredients, blending until smooth. In a jar, layer yogurt and cinnamon with smoothie mixture. Top with additional cinnamon. Enjoy!

#329 Spicy Mixed Greens Smoothie

122 Calories – 14g Carbs – 4g Fat – 7g Sugar – 3.5 Protein

Juice of 1 lemon, dash of cayenne pepper, 1 T ground flax seed, 1 T raw honey, 1 T peeled ginger root, ½ avocado, ¼ C frozen mixed berries, 1 C mixed greens 1.5 Cs dairy free milk.

Blend everything together until combined and frothy.

#330 The Cleanser Smoothie

118 Calories – 12g Carbs – 3g Fat – 4g Sugar – 3g Protein

Juice of 1 lemon, dash of cinnamon, ¼ t turmeric, ½ C cilantro, ½ C frozen mixed berries, 1 C mixed greens, 1.5 C dairy free milk.

Blend all ingredients together until combined and frothy in texture.

#331 Immune Boost Smoothie

111 Calories – 10g Carbs – 4g Fat – 5g Sugar – 1g Protein

3 drops stevia, 1 T ginger root, ½ red pepper, ½ C parsley, 1 C kale, 1.5 Cs dairy free milk.

Incorporate ingredients together until smooth.

#332 Liver Cleanse Smoothie

113 Calories – 11g Carbs – 2g Fat – 3g Sugar – 1g Protein

1-2 dashes of cayenne, ½ peeled grapefruit, 1 radish, 3 dandelion leaves, ½ C parsley, 1 C spinach, 1.5 Cs dairy free milk.

Combine until smooth.

#333 Savory Wake Up Green Smoothie

122 Calories – 15g Carbs – 4g Fat – 1g Sugar – 2g Protein

1-2 handfuls ice, 1-2 pinches cayenne pepper, ¾ t sea salt, 1 clove peeled garlic, 1 peeled lime, 1 peeled avocado, ½ chopped cucumber, 1 chopped carrot, 1 chopped tomato, 1 C chopped romaine lettuce, ¾ raw coconut water.

Blend ingredients until combined and smooth.

#334 Spicy Plum Green Smoothie

143 Calories – 12g Carbs – 2g Fat – 4g Sugar – 1g Protein

¼ t cayenne pepper, 1 t ginger, ½ t vanilla extract, ½ C soaked dates, 1 C oats, 1 C spinach, 1 frozen banana, 8 plums, 2 Cs almond or soy milk.
Blend together until creamy.

#335 Spicy Jalapeño Cilantro Green Smoothie

81 Calories – 20g Carbs – 1g Fat – 2g Sugar – 1g Protein

1 C ice, 1 C water, ½ seeded jalapeño, 5 sprigs cilantro, ½ juiced lime, 1 chopped cucumber, 1 chopped apple of choice, 1-2 handfuls kale.
Blend until smooth or it is desired consistency.

#336 Spicy Ginger Snap Green Smoothie

160 Calories – 37g Carbs – 2g Fat – 6g Sugar – 3g Protein

1 C ice, 1 C water, 1 T raisins, 1 T chia seeds, ½ inch ginger root, ½ t cinnamon, 1 chopped pear, 1 peeled orange, ½ C kale.
Blend until smooth and frothy.

#337 Spicy Pineapple with Cayenne Green Smoothie

105 Calories – 23g Carbs – 2g Fat – 12g Sugar – 2g Protein

1 C ice, 1 C water, 1 T chia seeds, 1-2 pinches cayenne, 1 juiced lime, 1 chopped apple of choice, ½ C frozen pineapple, 1-2 handfuls Swiss chard.
Combine all ingredients in a blender on high speed until combined and smooth.

#338 Ginger Banana Green Smoothie

124 Calories – 25g Carbs – 12g Sugar – 2g Fat – 4g Protein

1 T chia seeds, 2 handfuls ice, ½ C + extra unsweetened vanilla almond milk, ½ t cinnamon, ½-1 t ground ginger, 2 handfuls spinach, 1 frozen banana.
Blend until smooth. Top with additional chia seeds. Add more almond milk to achieve desired consistency if needed.

#339 Raspberry Jalapeño Smoothie

125 Calories – 22g Carbs – 3g Fat – 17g Sugar – 3g Protein

1 C ice, 1 C coconut water, 1 T hemp seed, ½ juiced lemon, ½ seeded jalapeño, 1 chopped apple of choice, ¼ C frozen raspberries, ½ C beets.
Combine ingredients until you achieve a smooth texture and deep red hued smoothie.

#340 Pear Ginger Lime Green Smoothie

114 Calories – 20g Carbs – 2g Fat – 15g Sugar – 2g Protein

Splash of coconut water, 1 lime, 1 t freshly chopped ginger, 1 Bartlett pear, 1.5 Cs spinach leaves, 1 C frozen mango chunks.

Blend ingredients together until smooth.

#341 Spicy BLT Bloody Mary Green Smoothie

257 Calories – 32g Carbs – 9g Fat – 13g Sugar – 8g Protein

Salt (to taste), 1 C vodka, ice, 2 t horseradish, 1 quartered jalapeño, 2 t Worcestershire sauce, 2 juiced limes, ½ C chopped cucumber, 2 T parsley, 2 T red wine vinegar, 4 Cs green tomatoes, ½ C baby spinach.

Combine ingredients until smooth and frothy. Garnish with a lemon wedge, romaine lettuce heart leaves, cherry tomatoes and crispy bacon.

#342 Spicy Mango Tango Green Smoothie

167 Calories – 28g Carbs – 6g Fat – 11g Sugar – 6g Protein

Handful ice, 1 T chia seeds, ½-1 C water, ¼-1/2 C fresh spinach leaves, ½ C frozen mango chunks, ½ C frozen banana.

Combine until mixture is your desired consistency. Top with additional chia seeds if desired.

#343 Sweet and Spicy Balancing Detox Smoothie

113 Calories – 18g Carbs – 4g Fat – 1g Sugar – 4g Protein

1.5-4 Cs ice cold water, 1 t raw honey, 2 pinches cayenne pepper, ½ juiced lemon, 1 apple of choice, 1 pear, 2 lacinato kale leaves, 1 C turnip greens, 1 T ginger root, ½ C spicy sprouts.

Blend until smooth. Top with a banana slice.

#344 Spicy Radish Smoothie

175 Calories – 21g Carbs – 3g Fat – 0.5g Sugar – 5g Protein

½ C orange juice, 1 C plain Greek yogurt, 2 T lemon juice, 1 C frozen strawberries, 1 C chopped carrots, 1 C raw radishes, 1 C spinach.

Blend until frothy.

#345 Spicy Vegetable Greeny

146 Calories – 20g Carbs – 6g Fat – 2g Sugar – 7g Protein

Handful ice, 1-2 pinches cayenne pepper, 2 cloves of garlic, 1 avocado, 1 chopped cucumber, 1 chopped carrot, and 1 C coconut water, 1 tomato of choice, 2 Cs romaine lettuce or spinach.

Combine components of smoothie until smooth.

#346 Spicy Tomato Gazpacho Grab Smoothie

205 Calories – 21g Carbs – 4g Fat – 2g Sugar – 10g Protein

1 C ice, pinch of red pepper flakes, 1/8 t ground black pepper, ¾ t sea salt, 1 T finely chipped red onion, 2 T finely chopped cilantro, 2 T fresh lime juice, ½ avocado, ½ cucumber, ½ red bell pepper, 2 chopped tomatoes of choice., 1 t jalapeño, ¼ t grated lime zest, ½ C spinach.

Blend all ingredients together until mixture is nice and frothy.

Chapter 13: Green Sweet Tooth

#347 Chocolate Peanut Butter Green Smoothie

322 Calories – 20.1g Carbs – 9.1g Fat - 13.3g Sugar – 22.9g Protein

4 Cs frozen greens of choice, ½ frozen banana, 1 T powdered peanut butter, 1 T unsweetened cocoa powder, 1 T chocolate protein powder, and 1.25 Cs unsweetened almond milk.

Blend all ingredients until smooth.

#348 Cacao Almond Green Smoothie

287 Calories – 9.3g Carbs – 4.9g Fat – 14.3g Sugar – 7.3g Protein

1 T maple syrup, 2 T cacao nibs, ¼ C almonds, 1 C almond milk, ½ frozen banana, 2 Cs kale.

Blend ingredients on high until combined.Serve with topping of cacao nibs.

#349 Dark Chocolate and Banana Green Smoothie

323 Calories – 12.3g Carbs – 9g Fat – 18.4g Sugar – 11.3g Protein

1 C spinach, 1 banana, 1 C almond milk, 3 T chia seeds, 2 T cocoa powder, ½ t vanilla extract.

Blend ingredients until smooth yet thick in texture.

#350 Creamy and Craveable Cacao Zucchini

190 Calories – 25g Carbs – 0g Fat – 9g Sugar – 5g Protein

1 C ice, 1 C vanilla almond milk, 1 t cinnamon, 1 T sunflower seed butter, 1 T cacao powder, 1 chopped zucchini.

Blend all ingredients until achievement of consistency you desire.

#351 German Chocolate Cake Green Smoothie

316 calories – 54g Carbs – 12g Fat- 25g Sugar – 6g Protein

1 C ice, 1 C water, ½ t cinnamon, 1 packet of Daily Good-Chocolate Blend, 1 T cacao powder, ¼ C pecans, 1 banana, 2 chopped pears, 1 handful beet greens, 1 C spinach.

Blend all components of smoothie until thoroughly combined, scraping jar as you go. Top with walnuts if desired!

#352 Peanut Butter C Smoothie

153 Calories – 28g Carbs – 5g Fat – 18g Sugar – 4g Protein

1 C ice, 1 C vanilla almond milk, 1 T peanut butter, 1 T carob powder, 1 T cocoa powder, 1 chopped pear, 2 handfuls chard.

Blend until completely combined. Top with sugar free caramel syrup/sauce.

#353 Sweet Potato Apple Bake Smoothie

297 Calories – 55g Carbs – 10g Fat – 36g Sugar – 2g Protein

1 C ice, 1 C water, 1 t baobab powder, ¼ t allspice, 2 dates, ¼ C pecans, 1 chopped empire apple, 1 C fingerling yams, ½ C kale.

Blend ingredients together to create a liquefied version of this famous dessert! Top with cinnamon or cocoa powder to serve.

#354 Caramel Apple Smoothie

143 Calories – 17g Carbs – 6g Fat – 10g Sugar – 5g Protein

1 C ice, 1 C water, ¼ C raw cashews, 1 t lucuma powder, 1 chopped apple of choice, 2 handfuls baby spinach.

Blend ingredients together to whip up a healthier version of a favorite fall treat!

#355 Cinnamon Apple Pie Smoothie

198 Calories – 30g Carbs – 11g Fat -16g Sugar – 3g Protein

1 C ice, 1 C water, 1 t acai powder, ½ t cinnamon, ½ t allspice, ¼ C raw walnuts, 2 chopped apples of choice, 1-2 handfuls fizz kale.

Blend components of this recipe to make a fresh C of a great tasting dessert!

#356 Pecan Pie Green Smoothie

228 Calories – 34g Carbs – 12g Fat – 18g Sugar – 3g Protein

1 C ice, 1 C vanilla almond milk, ½ T blackstrap molasses, ½ t nutmeg, ½ t cinnamon, ¼ C pecans, ½ C grapes of choice, 1 chopped pear, 1-2 handfuls baby spinach.

Blend ingredients to create a feel and taste-good experience from the fall season!

#357 Pumpkin Pie Smoothie

243 Calories – 43g Carbs – 11.2g Fat – 20g Sugar – 24g Protein

1 C ice, 1 t vanilla extract, ½ C light coconut milk, 1 T pumpkin pie spice, 1 scoop vanilla protein powder, ½ frozen banana, 1 C pumpkin puree, ½ C water, 1 handful baby kale.

Combine everything in a blender on high speed until mixture turns out creamy.

#358 5-Ingredient Chocolate Almond Chia Smoothie

198 Calories – 32g Carbs – 12.9g Fat – 13g Sugar – 5g Protein

2 T chia seeds, 2 T almond butter, 1 C baby spinach leaves, 1.5 Cs chocolate almond milk, 1.5 frozen bananas.

Blend until smooth in texture. Sprinkle with chia seeds if you choose.

#359 Healthy Shamrock Smoothie

223 Calories – 49g Carbs – 18g Fat – 12g Sugar – 6.9g Protein

8 mint leaves, ½ avocado, 1 frozen banana, 1 C spinach, 2.5 C non-dairy milk, 1 T honey or maple syrup.

Blend until smooth. Top with sugar free whipped cream, cacao nibs and/or mint leaves if desired. Enjoy!

#360 Chocolate Chia Smoothie

256 Calories – 34g Carbs – 14.4g Fat – 17g Sugar – 3g Protein

½ t vanilla extract, 2 T unsweetened cocoa powder, 3 T chia seeds, 1 C almond milk, 1 C ice, 1 C fresh spinach, 1 frozen banana.

Combine all ingredients together in a blender until nice and smooth. Top with sprinkle of cacao nibs if desired.

#361 Black Forest Antioxidant Smoothie

222 Calories – 23g Carbs – 12.2g Fat – 9.5g Sugar – 2g Protein

2 T coconut cream, 1 C baby spinach, 3 dates, 1-2 T unsweetened cocoa powder, 1 C frozen cherries, 1 t vanilla extract, ¾ C almond milk, 1 T flax seeds, ¼ C raw almonds.

Blend ingredients on high speed until you reach a creamy consistency.

#362 Key Lime Pie Smoothie

275 Calories – 39g Carbs – 18g Fat – 12g Sugar – 4.2g Protein

2 handfuls ice, 3 dates, 1-2 handfuls spinach leaves, ¼ C shredded coconut, ½ avocado, ¼ C freshly squeezed lime juice, 2 Cs coconut water.

Incorporate all ingredients together until blended well. Top with additional shredded coconut.

#363 Carrot Cake Smoothie

257 Calories – 23g Carbs – 11g Fat – 5g Sugar – 2g Protein

Dash of cinnamon, dash of nutmeg, 1-2 T chia seeds, ½ C frozen pineapple chunks, 1 frozen banana, ¼ C unsweetened coconut or almond milk, 3-5 juiced carrots, 2-3 handfuls baby spinach.

Blend components together until smooth. Top with additional cinnamon.

#364 Chocolate Covered Strawberry Shake

245 Calories – 30g Carbs – 12g Fat – 12.7g Sugar – 1.7g Protein

Handful ice, 1 T cacao powder, ½ t vanilla extract, 2 handfuls baby spinach. ¼ ripe avocado, 1 C frozen strawberries, 1 frozen banana, 1 C water or almond milk.

Combine ingredients until smooth. Add more ice if you want a thicker smoothie.

#365 Thin Mint Green Smoothie

230 Calories – 34g Carbs – 11g Fat – 14g Sugar – 22g Protein

1/8 t peppermint extract, ¼ C rolled oats, 1 scoop chocolate protein powder, 1 C frozen or fresh spinach, 1 C almond milk.

Blend until creamy. Top with additional mint.